The International Libra

THE GROWING CHILD AND ITS PROBLEMS

Founded by C. K. Ogden

The International Library of Psychology

DEVELOPMENTAL PSYCHOLOGY
In 32 Volumes

THE GROWING CHILD AND ITS PROBLEMS

Edited by EMANUEL MILLER

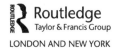
Routledge
Taylor & Francis Group

LONDON AND NEW YORK

First published in 1937 by
Routledge, Trench, Trubner & Co., Ltd.

Reprinted 2002 by
Routledge
2 Park Square, Milton Park, Abingdon, Oxon, OX14 4RN
Simultaneously published in the USA and Canada by Routledge
711 Third Avenue, New York, NY 10017
Transferred to Digital Printing 2007
Routledge is an imprint of the Taylor & Francis Group
First issued in paperback 2013

British Library Cataloguing in Publication Data
A CIP catalogue record for this book
is available from the British Library

The Growing Child and its Problems
ISBN 978-0-415-20997-7 (hbk)
ISBN 978-0-415-86443-5 (pbk)

CONTENTS

INTRODUCTION

THE object of this volume of essays is to provide insight into problems presented by the mental growth of children from five years of age to the close of adolescence. It is also hoped that guidance, too, will be obtained in steering children through the difficulties encountered in these years when school life begins and presents to the child special stresses.

It will be clear to most students of child development that by the time the fifth year is reached many conflicts have been created. The ties which bind mother and child during the period of suckling and weaning are strands in the fabric of character, and the love and hostility engendered by early family relations are so entangled with prohibitions that the personality is fundamentally shaped. So much so that parents having forgotten their own childhood stand bewildered before the questions, soliloquies and behaviour peculiarities of their young children. The common cry—" He will grow out of them ", is little more than a pious hope that the child will accept the principles of conduct which the adults have themselves adopted long ago. Unconsciously the parents behave towards their children as if the children must accept adult standards and the sooner the better. While we to-day adopt a more understanding view of the pace with which the child's adaptation can take place, we too are anxious to do all we can to " civilize " the child. We send them early to nursery schools, to socialize them, to get their sharp corners rounded off by contact with other children. But the parents cannot, in their anxiety, allow themselves to saddle others with the responsibility for moulding the mind and shaping behaviour. They must realize that as the child grows it does not entirely grow *away from* the emotional problems of the first five years. Teachers, governesses, and the like take over the rôle of parents in some measure, and however much the child may, at this stage, have achieved sufficient sense of reality to see such persons as what they are in themselves, it still responds to them in emotional situations with the same set of values with which they approached or were met by their parents. Parents must, therefore, expect that their children still have them in mind and that any conflicts which came into being as regards their relationship to their children will appear again in the child-teacher relationship.

Fortunately for most cases, unfortunately for others, by the time the child reaches its fifth year, it has settled the major problem of its relationship to its parents. This settlement, however, is not always as complete as external behaviour would lead us to believe. The settlement is frequently of the nature of an abdication of love and hostility motives, and yet not always an abdication of desires, but an unconscious pact of non-aggression, or perhaps a state of suspended hostility, an assumed neutrality, as the recrudescence of trouble at puberty clearly indicates.

It is for this reason that the period of quiescence, or latency as it is called, is so misleading both to understanding and in guidance of the child. It is of course true enough the larger number of children have by five sufficiently organized their lives to make a working adjustment to school life. They have matured by contact with reality, and benevolent parents, sufficiently well to see facts and persons without overwhelming emotional bias. They have largely accepted with equanimity parental control by absorbing benignly the personality of the parents, so that the edicts of conduct now become their *own* edicts, in the same way as a patient in post-hypnotic suggestibility believes he has himself willed and initiated the acts he performs under the suggestion of the therapist.

Another analogy is by no means a stretched one. A child that loves its parents finds it easier to accept their fiat, as the patient, respecting and almost loving the therapist, accepts uncritically his suggestions. For good development in the formative years, love, common sense and respect work together in producing adaptability. It means that rational satisfaction obtained from steady and respected parents becomes the foundation, not only of future social acquiescence, but freedom to enjoy the world of things and persons without a load of resentment, dissatisfaction and fear.

Perfection in adaptation can nowhere be found,

however. Evolution would have been arrested if complete harmony existed in primeval times between amœba and its environment. And furthermore, the very push and drive of life probably made the amœba too big for its boots, as it were. There is no standing still where life is concerned—it is always either forward or back. The child too can slip back, and we know only too well that when the child leaves home for the first time to go to school, he will, if free and growing like a plant turned towards the sun, eagerly enrich himself with the opportunity afforded him to learn more and to do more. When freedom at this age has not been achieved, if the child has remained fearfully dependent, or resentfully hostile, he will retire from the hostile new world of unfamiliar forces and unpredictable people, and he may respond by recoiling into earlier ways of obtaining satisfaction. He may even retire sullenly or fearfully into inaction or negativism, giving perhaps the appearance of a shorn lamb or of a blunted intelligence.

By the time the child has a more or less adult use of language it can deal with its world, not only by giving names to things, but by some measure of abstract thinking which makes the child more and more accessible to an adult mind. You now feel that you ought to be able to reason with him, and if you cannot, you feel bewildered and conclude that the child is either perverse or is too stupid to understand. Language, therefore, may actually stand between you and the child's emotional problem. Under the veneer of intelligence, which operates satisfactorily at moments when the child is unembarrassed, there is still the active life of instinct, which may have remained unsatisfied and dammed up because of a fear that its resurgence may lead to fearful consequences.

In the very young the imagination or fantasy of the child informs every thought and act which can be expressed in the child's play language which the understanding person can interpret. But the light of common day experience renders pallid this bright imaginative activity ; language disguises it and confines it to abstract terms ; and repressions have further relegated this fantasy life to the recesses of the mind where it proliferates, only rising to the top soil of consciousness in disguised ways. By this time the child, almost like the adult, becomes unaware of its own secret life, as it were, and as the claims of social life in home and school present to the child more and more of a manageable reality, inner motives of conduct become increasingly inaccessible to the observer. Even if the skilled understand, from behaviour, the hidden roots, it is not easy to appeal to the child unless the child himself by some technique is able to realize the connection between his acts and his motives. The latency period, therefore, presents problems which are hard to understand and still more difficult to handle, for at this stage parent, teacher and physician are dealing with neither a child nor an adult. The parent may feel himself in a no-man's land, sniped here by babyish passions and here startled by rational attacks which seem at times unanswerable. We can only enter the kingdom of the young mind by being as little children ourselves, equipped with their vocabulary, which means an understanding of the nature of their early impulses and of their fantasies. Understanding produces tolerance, and tolerance gives us the power to guide.

It is as imperative to handle wisely the child who is growing up as it is to guide the love and aggression of the young child before the age of five. While the child is still under the age of five, we are prepared to make concessions and to accept the child as new to the world and therefore with excusable instincts, but after this period modern society has ordained that the child must enter school, mix with his fellows and learn to use those intellectual instruments which will make him not only a fellow member in a community but an intelligent and productive one. Now when the child begins to use language intelligently, we are apt to conclude that it should be able to guide its own desires and impulses intelligently. This is, of course, a fallacy, for it is clear to any student of the child mind that abdication of instinctual rights has not been achieved by a signature. Most children's inner control of their passions is little more than a temporary pact of non-aggression. Deeper study teaches us that they are still well armed against us and their apparent quiescence is merely an armed neutrality. Those who guide children who are growing up may not be called upon to watch for every shade of behaviour which signalizes a remote emotional difficulty, but they must be prepared to have some insight into those red lights in behaviour which suggest that there is somewhere a hold-up in the mental traffic. The essays in this book attempt to bring to the general and special reader the sort of mild disorders which tell us that the child is troubled or maladjusted; and each writer will attempt to show how best to meet these difficulties, so that children may enter adult life on a path which has been cleared for them by the benevolent insight of those who guide them.

EMANUEL MILLER.

I. THE CHILD'S NEEDS AND HIS PLAY

By GWEN E. CHESTERS, B.A., INSTITUTE OF
MEDICAL PSYCHOLOGY

I. THE CHILD'S NEEDS AND HIS PLAY

BY GWEN E. CHESTERS, B.A., INSTITUTE OF
MEDICAL PSYCHOLOGY

CHILDREN play the world over. We have all played and we still play; perhaps it is this very universality and constancy of play which makes it possible for us to overlook much of its significance. Deprived of play we should be hardly better off than the proverbial fish out of water. We may not play by active movement; we may not mean to play at all; but we do play, if only in thought. Play should not be regarded as waste of time, or even as a means of merely passing time. It is more than purposeless activity. The effect of " too much " play has often been feared. It has been said that " if boys play when they are boys, they will play when they are men ", and, indeed, it is to be hoped they will, though not in the way implied in the saying. Through fear of its effects, play is sometimes curtailed, in a genuine if mistaken effort to encourage hard workers and a serious outlook on life. The results of such curtailment are often exactly the opposite to those intended.

It has long been recognized that :

> All work and no play
> Make Jack a dull boy,

3

yet, though we condone his weakness, we have a feeling that Jack is none the less weak to need to play. Jack's work, however, rests to a great extent on his play, and his play, as spontaneous, non-directed activity, has a function peculiar to it. Play is the means by which we make good needs not satisfied in any other way. We are to a great extent controlled by our needs, and it is in playing that we relieve many of the stresses we experience, almost without realizing that we are doing so. Through play we preserve our balance emotionally, free ourselves of the domination of primitive tendencies and so become capable of more developed interests and happy social relationships.

Though play is part and parcel of our life, it is by no means certain that at the present time all children have the sort of play they need. Under the usual conditions of modern life it is easy for the child's play to be inadequate for his needs. There is nothing artificial about good play, and natural surroundings always provide the means for it, however undeveloped these may be. If we were more primitive, we could perhaps afford to give less thought to provision for play, but in becoming to some extent civilized we have unwittingly allowed ourselves to be deprived of elemental play material, and, not realizing its significance, we have provided faulty substitutes for it. Many children have little contact with natural things, not enough space in which to play, and not enough natural material to play with. Even children who may have such opportunities can often make only restricted use of them. They have to be too clean and to play in too tidy a way. They

4

may have elaborate toys, but these are not always the boon they seem, and are poor compensations for the lack of plentiful natural material. It is not possible for us all to live where there is free space with its wealth of play material, but there is a lot we can do to minimize the disadvantage. There is much material within reach of all of us which can meet the child's needs and support his spontaneous development.

If we are to understand the function of his play and how best to provide for it at any stage, we must review briefly the child's general development and its relationship to his play. Play is related to the whole life of the child, it is not an isolated piece of behaviour. It shows some sequence as the child develops, but appropriate play cannot be regarded as rigidly determined by age. The sort of play suited to any particular child will depend upon his choice, which in its turn will depend largely on his previous experience and his general state, rather than on his chronological age. Hence successful play in adolescence will be determined by the satisfactoriness of earlier play, and it is therefore of great importance that the child's play life should be sound from the start. Play may be as much related to the past as to the present. Knowledge of his earlier development and requirements, and so perhaps of his deficiencies, will help us in making provision for him at any later stage. His play affects and is affected by his physical, intellectual, social and emotional development, and so as better to understand their general interdependence we will briefly discuss these four aspects of his life in relation to his play.

We will consider first his physical development. By the time he is five he has normally acquired good control of his body. He has progressed from the lying-down stage, through those of sitting-up, crawling, climbing and walking, and has at the same time gained skill in making many fine and specialized movements. He is very active, and the growing possibility of wider exploration and more skilled movement is a source of great satisfaction to him. Throughout the middle years of his childhood, just as earlier, much of his play tends towards, and in its turn is dependent upon, the development of his musculature, the perfecting of existing skills, and the acquiring of fresh ones. As he reaches adolescence his physical activity generally follows more special-ized lines, and more developed interest is added to his pleasure in general physical exercise.

Intellectually the child shows a similar inter-dependence of play and development. At five years he is aware of his separateness from other people and things. His world has gradually become organized. He knows himself and other people and objects as separate things, though he tends to give them meanings of his own. Many " real " things have for a long time some imaginary significance, but ultimately he separates the real from the imaginary. If progress has been smooth his interest has moved gradually from himself and his immediate concerns to other people and the objects of their interest, and then to similar and different things. All this has occurred largely through his play, where he has had social oppor-tunities of exploration and experimentation. His ingenuity and initiative have been roused and developed, and his interest, through finding a progressive outlet, is available for more cultural pursuits. The development of his speech has increased his possibility of interplay with other minds, and made more developed forms of play possible to him. All through his childhood he will learn from play, and continued exploration and experimenting will at the same time satisfy and maintain his curiosity. As his more primitive interests are satisfied, and his feelings given adequate outlet, he becomes free to follow his genuine interests without over-strong emotional bias. As he grows up, the field of his knowledge widens, and he becomes increasingly able to solve the problems presented by the things round him. Supported by his growing intellectual satisfaction, he becomes more and more capable of sustained effort in the pursuit of his enquiries, and progresses towards a stable cultural level. Such development is spontaneous. We can help him by making provision for his curiosity, and we must be careful not to damp down his enthusiasm by limiting him to restricted and over-specialized lines of enquiry at an early age. At a time when orthodox learning tends to follow a rather artificially selected range of subjects, it is increasingly important that the child should find opportunity of making good the deficiency through ample free play in a sympathetic environment.

His social development up to five years makes many demands upon him. Gradually he progresses from absorption in himself, his mother and those most nearly surrounding him, to the gradual acceptance of more and more substitutes for his early relationships and the sharing of his interests with them. His play reflects his social progress. A very young child plays to a considerable extent within himself. He responds to the play of others, but lacks the capacity for making very active play advances to them. As he develops, his play makes demands on the attention of other people and he arranges his play in accordance with his needs. Then he begins to allow for other people's wishes in playing, till he can play in a more co-operative way. His interest is stimulated by being shared, while its centre moves from himself and his immediate concerns. This gradual extension of his interests and his social contacts will continue all through his childhood, and the fostering of it is one of the most important functions of his play. It is in play that he can find adequate companions in his contemporaries, form sound co-operative relationships with them, and pursue shared interests without undue dependence on other people. He is safeguarded against dislocations of feeling, and ultimately achieves good give-and-take social behaviour not only in his play but in all his activities.

The child's emotional life is bound up with his social, intellectual and physical life—they are of course all interrelated—and in reviewing them we have already in part considered his emotional life. There can be no rigid definition of a child's emotional life at the age of five, but some things are true of him then as at any age. A child is potentially as happy and good as he is miserable and bad, and it is more normal for him to grow up happy and good than otherwise. A baby shows responsive, friendly feeling, confidence in those around him, great initiative, cheerful persistence when confronted with some obstacle, and much pleasure in activity and achievement. He also shows anger, anxiety, fear and grief in unduly difficult situations, and in these he appeals for help and comfort. A child has little control of his real situation, and little general understanding of it, and sometimes everyday circumstances or our own lack of insight increase the difficulty. But normally his happiness and confidence are preserved, and his unpleasant feelings reduced, as he has sympathetic handling and opportunity for the development of his own understanding and tolerance of the situation. Through play his pleasure and trust in life are maintained, and his capacity for meeting his experiences with sane and confident optimism develops. There are, however, many problems liable to disturb the child as he grows up, and here again his play is of the greatest importance. Children experience nursing, feeding, and cleanliness training, and these experiences are frequently associated with disturbed feeling, which persists when the actual circumstance with which it was connected has ceased to exist. There are also problems of thwarted activity, of lessening dependence on others, of family and social relationships, and of sexual development, each of them invested with feeling needing relief. The child's general balance is easily disturbed and his mental health depends upon its progressive restoration. In play he can express and find some solution of his

9

problems. His phantasies are played out and his feelings relieved. His most valuable and variable means of maintaining his confidence and happiness, of meeting the strains and stresses he experiences, and of helping forward his own development is play, and this holds good for play at any age.

We have seen that play has a varied function for the child, and it may make the basis of our provision for him clearer if we summarize briefly our conclusions. In play he can exercise and gain control of his body ; his interest is stimulated, satisfied and widened ; his social feeling built up ; his happiness maintained, and his feelings balanced. Without adequate play his needs remain unmet, and faulty and retarded development results. We can now consider how best we may provide for him, and we must bear in mind that this means both social and material provision. It will be simpler to consider these two aspects separately, though in practice there is no such division.

The child's social problem is the modification without dislocation of his early relationship to his mother, and he can be greatly helped in its solution through his play. He cannot be satisfactorily forced away from his mother, but she herself can help him to accept other interests by presenting him with them. His friendliness for her can be sustained, while his feeling and interest are spread from her to things she is doing, to other people round her, and to the things they are doing. His dependence on her alone lessens as he finds friendliness in other people and accepts them happily, and it is on a play level that social development can most easily be fostered. Failure to meet his need at an early age will make him over-demanding of attention later, and it is more difficult to satisfy him then than at the right time. An infant is largely dependent on others for his play. He needs play with other minds in a form in which he can take part. That is to say, he depends at this early age on other people's active play with him, as later he will need and enjoy play with them on a more intellectual level, either directly in talk, or more indirectly in reading, music and art. Most of us play intuitively or unwittingly with a small baby, by giving him freedom of movement, and time to enjoy his bath ; by talking to him as we bath, dress and feed him, and generally attend to his needs ; by showing him brightly coloured and moving things and putting him where he can see them, and in many other ways. It must not be supposed that such play on our part is trivial or unnecessary. It is in this way that the infant's contact with his mother is developed yet preserved, as he is given means of extending his interest. When he can sit up, he will enjoy being where household and outdoor work are being done and he should be talked to and not ignored as if he had " no mind ". When he can crawl and walk he will take a more active part in joining in the work, and this for him is play. A fifteen-months-old baby will make his " dinner " in a saucepan, " polish floors ", and " dig ". A small child needs early opportunity of finding pleasure in varied companionship, and it is good for him to play where there are other children, at first rather older than himself and more socially developed. He will soon be found to be imitating their play, and his contact with others is thus further strengthened and the sphere of his interest widened.   The age at which a child plays happily with other children depends very much on his experience of them, but his social development will be smoother if he has an opportunity of being with them from a quite early age.   He needs the companionship of his contemporaries to help him relinquish his mother without resentment, particularly if he is followed by other babies in his family. His emotional stresses are also greatly eased by his having other children to join in his dramatic and make-believe play, and their presence saves him from becoming too much engrossed in his own phantasies.   By the time he is five he should play happily with other children.   If he is found towards this age to be still very demanding of adult attention, lacking in interest, unwilling to play with other children or unusually hostile to them, he is needing play in some setting other than his usual.   Many nursery schools are run on play lines, and here the child has the needed support of a friendly adult as he makes and strengthens his contacts with other children.   From the age of five onwards he increasingly enjoys the companionship of other children.   Playing in " gangs " is a normal and spontaneous form of play from the age of six or seven onwards, and is one of the ways in which the child establishes his feeling of oneness with other children, and finds support for his growing social feeling, and for the development of socially directed independence.   With other children the child can play and invent innumerable group games, achieving at the same time a sound co-operative relationship with his fellows and a truer sense of proportion. The development of a ready sense of humour depends also to a great extent on the child's opportunities for play with other children. Throughout his childhood and his youth he needs other boys and girls with whom to play and with whom to share interests, while he must feel that the grown-ups in his immediate circle are genuine, disinterested companions who can appreciate and share his activities without forcing these along their own lines, and yet will let him share their interests as he is able. In playing with him they must let him take the initiative, and be content to follow his lead.

In addition to playing with the child, adults have a rôle seemingly more apart from, yet having a direct bearing upon his play, and if they fail to fulfil this rôle the child's play and general progress will inevitably be hampered. While they meet his social and emotional needs, they must give him the necessary intellectual support. The child has many questions which his contemporaries are no better able to answer than he is, and if he lacks necessary explanations his phantasy solutions will be unduly primitive and prolonged, and his play will be dominated by phantasy to the impeding of his exploration of reality. The child's body is an object of great interest to him, and at the same time a source of constant phantasy. He is concerned both with its structure, its " goodness " and its safety. Most children at some time ask questions about their bodies, but, whether they ask questions or not, they should be talked to about the body as a

PLAY CHART

The ages given are those at which material * should be introduced, but are only approximate.

Social Provision.	At all ages : Contemporary, and sympathetic adult companionship.
Free Material.	*Walking age or earlier :* Water, pots, funnels, rubber tubing, floating toys, scrubbing and cleaning materials, tea-sets. Dough. Sand and earth ; tray, pots, shovels. **15 months :** Chalk, paint, wood, paper. **3 years :** Crayons, pencils. **4 years :** Cooking materials, plasticine, garden and tools. **6 years :** Paints, household and camping equipment. *Adolescence :* Modelling, pottery, exhibitions.
Constructive Play.	*Up to 4 years :* Vessels with hole in top, pans with lids, jars with screw-caps, pegs with rings, peg-boards, bricks, wooden beads, hammering toys. **4 years :** Scissors, paste, mosaics, stitching cards. **5 years :** Wooden fitting toys, bricks, cardboard, wood, tools. stone, nails. **7 years :** Wool, canvas, material, weaving cards, small beads, knitting, crochet, puzzles, meccano. **12 years and onwards :** Making things to wear and use ; metal work, carving, various crafts, electrical and wireless apparatus.
Acting Play.	*Walking age :* Boxes, covers, sticks. **4 years :** Pieces of curtain and material, old finery, etc., grease paint. **6 years and onwards :** Puppets, plays, films.

Stories and Reading.	*Up to 5 years:* Nursery rhymes, picture books, short stories. *Adolescence:* Modern and earlier classics. Biography. Travel. Verse.	*6 years:* Fantastic and reality stories. True stories. Children's verse.	*9 years:* Adventure stories, mystery stories.
Physical Play.	*Up to 6 years:* Pulling and pushing toys, balls, stairs, step-ladder, swing, see-saw, tricycle, dancing, swimming, picnics.	*6 years:* Hoop, skipping-rope, bicycle, rowing, camping.	*9 years:* Organized games.
Musical Play.	*Up to 4 years:* Rattle, stick and tin, being sung to, bell, clapping games.	*4 years:* Drum, whistle, comb, mouth-organ, singing, eurythmics.	*8 years:* Learning an instrument. *9 years:* Wireless, Gramophone, Concerts: according to interest.
Social Games.	*Up to 9 years:* Skittles, tiddley winks, marbles, snap, ludo and simple board games.	*9 years and onwards:* Darts, quoits, bagatelle, card games, chess, billiards.	
Made Toys.	*Before 1 year:* Brightly coloured objects, cuddly toys, dolls. *12 years:* Electrical toys.	*Walking age and later:* Dolls' house, bed and pram, pets, wooden engines, small cars, steam-rollers, trolleys, cranes, aeroplanes, station and garage sets, popguns, bows and arrows, clockwork toys, Noah's ark, farmyard, wild animals, small figures.	

* The material suggested here for earlier ages should be available to the older child until he abandons it of his own accord.

matter of intellectual interest. His strong bones and supple joints with their general arrangement, the little " pipes " for blood and the holding of blood within tissue, how he breathes, what happens to food after it has gone into his mouth, and the fact that he " grows mended " after he has cut or hurt himself, are all matters from the understanding of which the child gains support for his developing curiosity and feeling of general confidence. Without understanding, he remains preoccupied. He is equally if not more interested in where he came from and how he was made, and if left unanswered these problems may arrest the all-round development of his play. There are also many questions about the things that he hears of and sees, and as his interest extends from his own concerns it must be satisfactorily met. The fuller meeting of it is for the most part inevitably left, under our present system, to his so-called education, but where this tends to be too specialized to serve the child's more general enquiries, a sympathetic hearing at home and the making available of the needed means of satisfaction, must make good the deficiency. The progress of his play to a level where difference in intellectual and emotional demand is one of quality not quantity, while it depends partly on the meeting of his emotional and social needs, is to some extent determined by the provision made for his intellectual development; and it rests largely with adults to help this intellectual balancing of his play.

The discussion of the provision of play material will, of necessity, seem more detailed, but the importance of the social aspect of play must not be lost sight of. Any material can serve as a basis of social play, while some, as we shall see later, is more particularly suited to it. As was suggested earlier, appropriate play material is not altogether age-determined. An attempt will consequently be made here to present it in sequence rather than to classify it according to age. The accompanying chart of play provision gives a rough age classification. Some children seem to play very little, or to use material in an irrelevant way, and this may be · because their supply of more primitive material has been inadequate. Sequence of material will therefore be of help in suggesting what earlier material might meet their need. Some children are found to be troublesome and " never out of mischief ", and they may be suffering or have suffered from a general lack of adequate material, and for such children earlier forms of provision are more necessary than those supposedly related to their age.

There are some kinds of play which can stand us in good stead throughout our lives, and though the forms of such play are of great variety, they will be found to be related to primitive kinds of activity. It will be these more permanent and consequently essential kinds of play with their modifications which will be first considered. They will, in the main, be found to be connected with play with free materials, with acting play, with physical play, with banging and " noise " play and with constructive play.

Play with crude materials will first be discussed together with the sequence of play to which it gives rise. These materials provide the child with the means of bridging the gap between his phantasy and reality play, for with such materials he can play according to the needs of his feelings, and at the same time explore and gain understanding of the possibilities of the material, with as much satisfaction in such exploration as in the expression of his phantasies. They help him in the levelling up of his mental development. His feelings are eased and modified, his activity stimulated, and his thought brought into play. A child needs to be able to express his destructive tendencies, and to relieve the underlying anger and anxiety, and crude materials meet this need as no other material can. The child can " ill treat " the material, or destroy what has been made, without doing real damage, and with the possibility of making again. Crude materials allow also for his need to make a mess and to clean up, with the relief of the related feelings and phantasies. He can use them, too, for genuine constructive play. The unifying effect of play with this sort of material helps forward his general mental organization. As his more primitive interests are satisfied and his thinking stimulated he moves towards a more skilled and cultured level of activity. Another feature to be noticed about these basic kinds of play is that they provide the child with a ready means of establishing and extending his social contacts, through the sharing of activity needed and enjoyed by all children. The interests to which such play give rise often continue into adult life, and give the child a lasting link with other minds.

Amongst our cruder materials water is placed first. It is a most valuable plaything, yet to many children it is a lost treasure. Beyond being washed and bathed they have little contact with it, and even washing and bath-time may be little more than business-like ceremonies. Yet water corresponds to some of the deepest and most primitive needs within the child. He can use it to meet persisting needs related to his early feeding and cleanliness training, yet put it to more developed uses and gain understanding of its behaviour. A young child often needs to let the taps run, dabble his hands in water and splash it. He will take pleasure in pouring it from one vessel to another, playing " tea-parties ", watering the garden, washing the floor, washing clothes, syphoning water through rubber tubing, and making harbours in a bowl or sand-tray. Material related to early water-play includes small vessels and funnels ; rubber tubing, floating toys and boats ; and scrubbing and washing materials. When the child has no streams or ponds in which to play, he has all the greater need of home provision. He is less likely to make a troublesome mess if he can play with water outdoors, and do also such jobs as watering the garden, but where this is not possible he should be allowed to play in the sink, and to join in when work requiring water is being done. He will also play many cleaning games of his own. Water-play is of importance in his general development, and children with feeding, speech, cleanliness-training and constipation difficulties often find it of great help. Children of any age like to play with water in some way, and such play, as it becomes free from emotional complications, can provide an abundant source of later activity. Where the child has access to outdoor water he will find valuable scope for his play, and his interest in it will link on to his pleasure in exercise and in watching the behaviour of living things.

Sand- and earth-play is similarly valuable for the child's feelings and ingenuity, and from making a mess, " pies " and " ice-cream ", he will pass to making castles, houses, " seasides " and other scenes, while the provision of tools and a piece of garden will further strengthen his contact with reality. For sand- and earth-play the child needs a tray (for indoor play), shovels, small pots, sweeping brushes, and later if possible a piece of garden and some tools. A good substitute for a sand-tray is an ordinary meat baking-tin, and flour-scoops make good sand-shovels. Where it is possible the child should have a sand-pit in the garden, and if he lives by the seaside should naturally spend as much time as possible on the beach. Earth- and sand-play also help feeding, cleanliness and speech problems, and free play with them, as with water, will save the child from making irrelevant use of more developed material, such as crayons and paints, when they are provided for him. He will be able to use these in a more purposeful way if his need to make a mess has been and still is being satisfied in other ways. His sand- and earth-play also brings him into contact with living things and their habits, giving him a further spread of interest from himself through insight into other manifestations of life, as he sees them in rooted things like plants, as well as in creatures which move about as he does.

Play with dough also gives the child support in

his solution of the problems related to his earlier experiences. Dough can be made for him by mixing flour and water. Eating difficulties, speech defects, constipation and cleanliness difficulties are often greatly relieved by play with this material. As experimental material, dough has many possibilities. It can be fingered, squeezed, flattened, spun out and shaped. The child will soon begin to make " cakes " and will want to cook them, and when he reaches this stage he should be given some simple materials which, unlike flour and water dough, will be eatable when cooked. He can be shown how to rub a little butter into the flour and, if he has a little sugar to add, this when mixed with water and cooked will make quite eatable biscuits. He very quickly learns to rub butter into the flour for himself. He will like, too, to stew fruit, and to cook potatoes, chestnuts and apples in the fire. This kind of play leads up, as does his other household and outdoor play, to his camping play, and this will be described later. It is of importance for the child's feeling of security that he should have some elementary knowledge of how his life is maintained, and some opportunity of providing food for himself.

Material related to household and outdoor work is of particular value, as in having the use of it the child gains insight into how his actual life is provided for, and his feeling of safety, and his confidence in life and himself are strengthened. For children who spend most of their time in the nursery and walking in the park, and later in a resident school, this aspect of things is of particular importance, if their contact with life in general is to be established. Provision must be made for them, if only in a " play " way, in making available opportunities of cleaning, cooking and gardening play open to children who have freer access to a kitchen and garden. All play related to household and garden occupations will be more enjoyed by the child if it can be done with a grown-up doing work of a similar kind. Most children will sometimes ask whether they may join in, and will find great pleasure in sharing the " work ". House play and camping play are related to this early life-maintaining play, and the provision of some boxes, sticks and old covers for making huts and tents, and later of a real tent, will meet it. Picnics and camping give great pleasure to the child, and fire-lighting should be allowed him. A child enjoys all such play throughout his childhood, and it is frequently continued into adult life. Contact with natural life is a rich source of intellectual interest to the child. In addition to learning about things which affect his own life he learns about other kinds of life and the conditions affecting them. His exploratory interest has its roots here, and this will be of value throughout his life. It does, however, need progressive satisfaction and the support of varied free play from the beginning, if it is to run freely along sound lines.

Having reviewed the durable forms of play related to cruder materials, we can now go on to other forms of gradually developing play which have a primitive basis. Clay and plasticine become of increasing value as the child's skill in manipulation grows, usually from the age of four onwards. As his interest moves towards the representing of a variety of definite things and situations he needs material of a more stable kind. His need for the very plastic material may still continue, and he should have plasticine in addition to, not as a substitute for, dough. Clay and plasticine serve as media for the most varied phantasies, which can thus find expression, relatively free from anxiety if they are of a destructive kind, and always with great satisfaction to the child. As his feelings find relief he will become more interested in the constructive possibilities of the material and his manipulative skill will increase. Plasticine can be had in many colours, but while the child is using it principally for the relief of his phantasies and feelings, it may be found that he mixes the colours together, and then, disliking the look of the material, plays little with it. In such cases it is better to give him plasticine of one colour, perhaps terra cotta, until he is interested as much in the way in which he can make things as in what he makes. Modelling play finds a more developed expression in adolescence and adult life in pottery making, modelling, sculpturing and carving.

Paper, chalk and paint should be available for children from an early age, as they provide at the same time a means of developing skill, and of expressing feelings and problems for which the child has no words. As his skill increases these materials can be supplemented by the addition of crayons and pencils. It is not desirable for the child to be taught at first how to draw and paint. He should be allowed to paint as he wishes, and representations of what looks more " real " should not be urged upon him. Neither should he be expected to draw his picture first and then paint it. In a similar way, plain paper is of more value to him than outline pictures to be copied, filled in or traced. He also needs such things as pieces of wood and boxes to paint. At first he will find more satisfaction in painting with his finger or a big brush and liquid paint mixed ready for him, than with a small brush and a paint-box. Cheap poster paint can now be bought, and this, if mixed with water in jars, will make an economical supply of paint. When his interest in how to paint shows itself spontaneously in experimentation, teaching of actual technique will be of value to him, but the cramping of his expressiveness must be guarded against. Painting and drawing can give the child lasting relief and pleasure as he grows up, and his interest in it will be extended to the work of other people. Such interest can be met by his seeing their work in books and at exhibitions, but this is best shared with his contemporaries or with some adult to whom such things give real pleasure, rather than with someone who makes a " dutiful " study of them. These and similar interests will give him much recreation in later life, and again they are of a kind which he can share with others.

Acting play provides the child with further valuable means of expression, and this is again a progressively developing form of play. Only simple material is needed—pieces of curtain and material, old finery, covers and discarded clothes. Early make-believe play, hardly realized by the child as such, develops into spontaneous dramatic play when the child knows that he is "pretending", and the provision of simple material specially related to it (from three years onwards) will help the child's freer expression of his feelings, and his distinction of reality from phantasy. He will be found to play many games related to his everyday experiences, his wishes and his relationships to other people. He needs these games to help him towards a truer balance of his feelings and finds great satisfaction in them, becoming better able to accept the situations of everyday life. The things around him in the house and outdoors, as well as his own toys and articles more particularly provided for it, are made to serve as media for his dramatic play. He often plays his "tucking-in" games in bed when he gets under the bed-clothes, or makes them into a tent, and he uses tablecloths and other covers draped over furniture for similar play. A clothes-horse or a step-ladder make a good foundation for an indoor tent. Other frequent acting games are tea-parties, trains, mothers and fathers, witches, fairies, school, policemen, soldiers, burglars, cowboys and Indians, fighting and killing, and many other more individual games. Stories are acted, at first when they coincide with the child's own phantasies, and it is only gradually that he becomes capable of more detached play, and of finding satisfaction in acting out less personally related scenes and plays. Home-made puppet shows give him a further means of acting as he needs. A specially made stage and puppets are not essential for this, for an adequate stage can be made of a table draped with a cloth, and puppets which can be made at home of strong cardboard, and then dressed, serve the child very well. In this way he can act quite freely scenes of his own invention. Though acting of this sort possibly makes less social demands on him than acting with other children, it may be of great help in easing his more personal disturbed feelings, and so it tends ultimately to help him socially. As his feelings are relieved and his thinking stimulated he will take pleasure in finding more and more apt forms of expression, with increasing interest in both reading and acting. He will also enjoy seeing films and plays. Young children do not need very frequent visits to films and plays if they have good scope for play elsewhere, but they enjoy seeing representations of what corresponds to their own phantasies or real experience. Children like plays similar in theme to the stories they enjoy, and these will be discussed later. The choice of films for young children is not easy, but Mickey Mouse, Shirley Temple, most funny films and Wild West films are popular with them. It is better that the older child should not see films presenting him with experiences and problems normally to be considered by him in later adolescence, particularly when he is still busy with many of his early problems, and there are many films of well-known stories and others of more balanced interest which will cater for him during adolescence. His own choice of films will, of course, to a great extent depend upon the general satisfactoriness of his own play and on the soundness of feeling in the people with whom he lives.

Connected with his pleasure in acting and watching others act, is his pleasure in being told stories, in being read to, and, later, in reading for himself. He takes part in the exploits of imaginary people of whom he reads, becoming progressively freer from strong emotional needs and more developed in his choice of stories. Children differ to some extent according to their needs in the sort of stories they enjoy, but there is a wide range of stories which most of them like. Little children prefer books with a picture on every page, and which describe the mischievous behaviour of some child or animal. There are many such animal stories from the small Tippeny Tuppeny books to the longer stories of the Beatrix Potter series and Dr. Dolittle. Small children prefer short stories which can be completed easily in one reading, and they should, when possible, sit on the lap of whoever is reading so that they can see the words. They will be found to ask spontaneously by the age of four and five such question as " Which word says ' piggie ' ? " and in this way their interest in reading for themselves is fostered. They should also sometimes be asked to tell the stories to whoever usually reads to them, or to someone else, so that they can experience the pleasure of contributing. In cases where reading difficulties occur, it is sometimes found that these are in part related to the child's pleasure in the social relationship involved in being read to, and it is therefore important that his general social life should be satisfactory, so that his need to monopolize attention may not make him unwilling to make the effort to read for himself. Some stories are partly enjoyed for their sound and among them are those which have similar phrases frequently repeated, as in " The Old Woman and her Pig ", the " Three Little Pigs ", " This is the House that Jack Built ", and similar stories. Nursery Rhymes remain favourites for a long time. Children of five and older like magic and fantastic stories found among the many fairy tales. They continue for a long time to like stories of children and of animals (the prototypes of children) of an imaginative yet possible kind. The stories chosen for them should have, from the child's point of view, a happy ending. By the time children begin to ask about stories, " Is it true ? " they will enjoy true stories of animals and of the lives of children. They will also like stories of imaginary people representative of reality. At this stage, fairy stories tend to be replaced by adventure and mystery stories, and the interest in these lasts for a long time. Stories with a pseudo-moral bias tending to intensify the child's feeling of guilt are to be avoided. The child's choice of reading in adolescence (and, of course, earlier) is likely to be the sounder for his having had opportunities of other expressive play. He will like stories of varied setting and character, and there are many such stories among the modern and older classics. He needs literature which can give him a balanced play of feeling without swamping his thinking, but his wish for stories in which the emotional interest is falsely exaggerated will depend very much on the general satisfactoriness of his other forms of recreation and of his social relationships. This will also influence his later choice of books and his power of critical appreciation, and will determine whether he will prefer only books which will meet his immediate emotional needs, or whether he will be able to enjoy books having a less subjective appeal. Only as a result of some degree of emotional detachment is he able to value a book for its intrinsic merits, and to find pleasure in it as a work of art. As he grows up, and the play of his intellect balances that of his emotions, he will read with true appreciation and judgment, and here again find a medium of friendly relationships with other people.

Play which allows freedom of movement and scope for bodily exercise is important at all ages. Just as a baby needs freedom for kicking, crawling, climbing and walking, older children need satisfaction in the exercise and control of their bodies. Pushing and pulling toys, balls, swings, see-saws, tricycles, hoops, skipping-ropes, stairs, step-ladders and trees all provide for early forms of exercise. Rhythmic movement and dancing also support the child's spontaneous tendencies, but care should be taken that his spontaneity of movement should not be hampered by too formal teaching. Given companionship, children will play innumerable running-about games, largely traditional or newly invented, and they find great reassurance and pleasure in such play. Children of nine years and onwards begin to find satisfaction in more organized forms of sport, and will often adopt them spontaneously, but they still need ordinary free opportunities of exercise. It is in games, as in household and garden work, that grown-ups can find a good opportunity of maintaining their contact with children, and children of further social development. In adolescence games can provide the child with great physical satisfaction and good social support, though the over-encouragement of competitive feeling frequently detracts from their value. There are some children to whom organized games seem to give little pleasure and no relief, and for such children it is important that they have plenty of contact with other children, and opportunities of freer forms of exercise such as swimming, walking, dancing or climbing. They will also probably find greater satisfaction in such activities as hiking and camping, where interest is not limited to exercise in itself. Physical play has also a ready carry-over into adult life in games, walking, climbing, dancing, swimming, rowing, skating and other forms of exercise.

Little children also need opportunities of making a noise, and their early rhythmic banging and chanting play can be developed along ultimately less disturbing and more social lines by the early provision of a drum or a tin on which to beat, a bell, a whistle, a comb and a mouth-organ. They enjoy listening to singing and being sung to, and as their pleasure in rhythm and musical sounds increases will become more capable of making the necessary effort to master the technique of playing some instrument, or of singing, in order to produce pleasurable sounds themselves. Listening to music can give them great satisfaction, and here again children and grown-ups can enjoy their pleasures, and the child find a further basis of lasting common interest with his contemporaries as he grows up and in adult life. Wireless and gramophones provide a ceaseless fund of music, but the choice of music listened to will again depend to a great extent on the adequacy of the child's other expressive play. Genuinely interested, appreciative and critical talk about the music heard will help him in his choice, but here too he is quick to detect dutiful efforts to "teach" him. Music should not be limited for him at an early age to these more mechanical devices, for they have disadvantages, to be discussed later, similar to those of complicated mechanical toys.

Play with more definitely constructive material has lasting interest. It becomes gradually more developed, and pleasure in it can be shared with others. It is of value, too, in helping the child to tolerate thwarting and frustration, as he learns to recognize and accept the limitations of his material. Such frustration has fewer implications for him than that which is imposed on him by older and stronger people ; it is impersonal, and leaves him free to experiment further, so that it helps him to accept more readily what is inevitable. If he recognizes inevitability as something which is in the nature of the situation, not as something forced on him from outside, his initiative will be directed towards solving real problems, rather than to circumventing authority. No distinction is made between material for boys and girls, as such a division is often artificial and small boys enjoy stitching just as girls enjoy hammering. Very little children already play constructive games, improving their manipulative skill frequently with accompanying phantasy satisfaction. Vessels with a hole in the top and something to drop into them, pans with lids, and jars with screw caps, pegs with rings, boards with holes in them and pegs that fit, beads to thread, mosaics, wooden bricks, hammering toys, scissors, paper, paste and stitching cards give the necessary early scope. Later material includes wooden fitting toys; stone bricks; cardboard; nails, wood and tools; puzzles; constructive toys like meccano; weaving cards and wool; beads, canvas and stuff; wool, crochet hooks and knitting needles. It is perhaps usual in later childhood and adolescence for girls to be interested in sewing and knitting, and boys in carpentry and in such constructive toys as meccano. But it will be found that some boys like knitting and many girls like woodwork, and such play should be made possible for them. We prefer men tailors, but we frequently laugh at younger boys who wish to sew or knit, and tell them " That's a girl's game ". Material such as cardboard, wood and cloth, which can be put to a variety of uses, are more important than more set constructive material. Children develop great initiative in their use of raw material, and at first are much more concerned with what they make than with how they make it. This early attitude to " work " should be accepted; for, as their skill increases with practice, they will become more interested in the quality of their work and in how to achieve the best results. Before they can do this, they must have opportunity of satisfying their need to make something for themselves. Children in adolescence frequently develop their constructive play along one or two special lines, and take great pleasure both in the quality of their work and the result achieved. Girls begin to find satisfaction in making attractive things to wear, and disturbed and developing feeling finds considerable relief and support in doing so. Boys also make really useful things for themselves; in following up their experimental needs they may become very skilled in making electrical and wireless apparatus, and in doing other household jobs. Carving and metal work provide other satisfying crafts for both boys and girls. These and other crafts, such as pottery, are not very easy to provide for at home, but there are good classes in most art and technical schools open to adolescents and older people. The making of things in common with his contemporaries is of great help socially to the adolescent, and helps him to achieve a more stable balance of interest and feeling. His emotional life has a wider basis if he and his friends can find pleasure in common activity as well as in their interest in one another.

More directly social play is found in the more set forms of children's games, and more developed forms of this sort of play also last into adult life. Early games which children much enjoy are skittles, tiddley winks, marbles, snap and the usual simple board games such as ludo and snakes and ladders, besides other games of their own invention, like " conkers ". These games help the child to accept order and justice, and as these are just part of the game he gains a more objective understanding of them than when his own idea of law and order is confused by his feelings towards the authorities who enforce them. When he is confronted by just demands of a more personal kind, he will be less likely to resent them as merely arbitrary if he has previously found such demands to be inherent in some more objective situation. Later games are provided by such material as darts, quoits, bagatelle and billiards, card games, draughts and chess. As he grows older the child should be provided with games making demands on his skill rather than with games whose result depends largely on chance. It is better for him, in the present competitive state of society, to learn to accept his own limitations, and to find satisfaction and security in the exercise of his skill in friendly surroundings, where the situation offers each an equal chance of success, than to have to fall back on games whose object is the outdoing of rivals by luck.

We must now pass to the more transitory but none the less important kinds of play. These are in the main less lasting because they are more nearly related to early individual phantasy, which fades as the child's contact with reality is strengthened. But if the child is to find due satisfaction in reality he must have the opportunity to play out his phantasies. As was mentioned before, he tends to be chiefly preoccupied with his early experiences, and he must find some solution of these problems if he is to be relatively free of them in later life. Real circumstances will inevitably seem difficult to him at times and he will tend to retreat from them. The necessary reassurance can be gained by material with which the child can act out his phantasy without losing contact with the reality situation, and in this way a retreat into day-dreams is prevented. An old clothes-basket or empty boxes can fill many parts in the child's play. Along with some old covers he will use them for his many "tucking-in" games which give him great satisfaction. Their adequacy can be increased by the provision of "cuddly" toys and dolls, so that child's play will be less centred on himself, and his games will become more developed. A doll's house and bed, which can if necessary be made easily for him from boxes, and a doll's pram, further extend his play and make it of more value to him. Children have many family and social problems with which to deal, and, while their understanding and control of real situations is limited, they need opportunities of externalizing their feelings and arranging things satisfactorily for themselves. Little children, both boys and girls, play family and school games, and with girls such games often continue up to the age of twelve and even beyond. Material for these games might well include pets, for the possession of a kitten or a puppy is a great reassurance to a child, and at the same time adds greatly to his pleasure in, and understanding of, living things. Other material having reference to similar developmental problems includes wooden engines, small steam-rollers, cars, trolleys and cranes, aeroplanes, and later clock-work toys. These meet the needs of both boys and girls, though it is usually boys who continue to play with them when girls are more occupied with dolls. Station and garage sets (made of lead) are good supplementary material.

The provision of mechanical toys is not essential

for early play, and presents of complicated electrical toys are best delayed until the child is capable of some understanding of the mechanism involved. Very young children see many events which they are inevitably at a loss to understand, and frequently think of as the outcome of some sort of magic. Experiences of this type in connection with play, and the continued presentation of problems which are beyond the child's intellectual powers of solving, can only tend to weaken normal curiosity; and to provide means of satisfying normal curiosity is part of the function of play. Thrown back on a more infantile form of explanation, children tend to revert to an infantile level of gratification, as other modes of finding satisfaction through greater effort are not yet securely established. They can enjoy without effort the inexplicable workings of the things round them, and will accept them in much the same way as they did earlier " magic " happenings. Not having sufficient opportunity of achieving sound satisfaction as a result of carrying their enquiries through to a logical end, they are left with the more infantile pleasure connected with magical (mechanical) happenings. It is in this possibility of preserving an effortless infantile satisfaction, that the blasé attitude of many " spoilt " children has its origin.

A Noah's Ark, a farmyard, wild animals and small figures (made of lead or wood) furnish the child with further varied means of expressing his ideas and feelings, and of developing his thoughts. The child must have opportunity of strengthening his good feeling and of representing his angry, bad feeling as outside himself, as well as of dealing with what he feels to be the dangerous elements in other people. He can do this by concrete representations, and so become able to tolerate the anxiety which accompanies his aggressive feelings. He can also reconcile his mixed feelings about his parents and others, by being able to take sides against the " bad ", and feeling that he has the support of what he recognizes as good. If he can find a satisfactory vent for his feelings in an indirect way, his real circumstances, with their inevitable thwartings, will put less of a strain on him, and intolerance of the " badness " of others will not lead him to reject them or over-idealize them. Tame and wild animals, toy soldiers and other figures serve a great variety of play along these lines. The advantage of having concrete material for the portrayal of the child's phantasies lies in the simultaneous stimulation of his interest. He is much less dominated by his feelings than he would be if he had no such means of dealing with them.

There are, of course, many more toys to be had than have been mentioned here, but an effort has been made to present what may be regarded as the more essential provisions for play. The meeting of the child's most common and urgent needs has been made the basis of selection, and provision for these is simple rather than elaborate. In choosing toys there has sometimes been a tendency to over-intellectualize play, and to substitute learning material for toys. This has often meant the restricting of freer play, or the provision of what is inadequate to the child's needs. Good play does teach

the child, and " improve his mind " in the widest
sense, and it does so without being turned into
unsatisfactory work. It is largely through play
that the child is enabled to make full use of his
intellectual capacity, and this freedom depends, as
we have seen, less on the so-called training of his
mind than on the balancing of his various needs.
A false work-element also tends to displace real
play in much organized sport, and as this is usually
of a competitive kind it thus loses the really social
and individually satisfying qualities of freer games.
We do not need to impose work on the child.
His spontaneous interest leads him towards exerting
effort to compass his ends. Having experienced in
his play the pleasure of achieving his aim through
such activity, he becomes capable of sustained activity and of waiting for results, without giving up
in face of difficulty. So he becomes able to do
what is ordinarily regarded as work. We shall
not help him to spontaneous sustained effort by
limiting his possibilities of more general satisfaction and endeavouring to develop his intellect more
than his emotions. Good work and developed
play have much in common, though in general
work can only be play of so intellectual a kind that
it can fulfil only one of the functions of play. Even
when work becomes, in adolescence and later life,
our most serious business, it is necessary that our
play life should continue. For many people, work
under present conditions can have little even of the
intellectual value of play, and it is to their leisure
that they look for most of their satisfaction. But
good use of leisure can best be made by people who

have a sound play history, for if they have had little or no access to earlier progressive means of satisfying their needs they will find little relief in more developed and acceptable forms of recreation, and will be unable to enjoy what otherwise might give them real pleasure. They will tend to resort to more primitive forms of amusement, or else may become people of few interests. Their social life will therefore be hampered, for they will have fewer means of contact with balanced people.

We have discussed earlier the social significance of play, and, however adequate our material provision may be, the child will still suffer if his *social* needs are not met. Without contemporary companionship he may be left too much to the pursuit of his personal phantasies, and lack the means of establishing his real interests through sharing activity with other children. His dependence upon grown-up attention will also be prolonged as he has insufficient substitutes for it. We cannot force him to independence without damaging him, but this will develop spontaneously through social play. To exact independence of him without providing him with companionship can only increase his feeling of insecurity. Adults are, however, of importance in his play, and, in addition to what has been noticed earlier as regards their part in it, something may be said here about the general attitude of adults to play. Children's play should in the main be accepted. It is normal for them to get dirty, and they should be dressed accordingly and not be expected to play too tidily. Criticism of play as silly or babyish is to be avoided. Should it appear so to us, the general scope of the child's play, social and material, should be looked into, for it is through attention to this, rather than through the effect of unfavourable comment, that the difficulty can be remedied. Some play, and the children's talk about it, may seem to grown-ups somewhat primitive, but such play is normal to young children, and can be accepted in a non-committal way by adults. Unsympathetic comment upon it is liable only to prolong it, and where children feel obliged to hide such play their feeling of guilt is increased, and their confident relationship with adults endangered. Play of this kind can be modified and developed by giving the necessary intellectual support to the child, as suggested earlier. Initiative and ingenuity are to be encouraged, though not over-stimulated, and discouragement through the expectation of too high a standard of achievement must be guarded against. Children find great reassurance in the companionship of friendly adults, and, while normal, happy children do not make undue demands on their attention, they do make suggestions of shared play and find great pleasure in it. In adolescence, when many of his contemporaries may be somewhat disturbed emotionally like the child himself, the need for steady, confident companionship is great, and friendly relationships and sharing interests with the adults round him, while they do not hamper his developing independence, give him the stability he needs.

We have seen that satisfactory play can lead us to freedom in our choice of recreation, and to the enjoyment of what is of worth in itself. It will also influence our choice of work, our attitude to it, and the way in which we do it. There are many possibilities before the child who has scope to explore and follow up his interests, and such opportunity is of great importance if he is to find what will call out spontaneous, renewed effort from him. The best work is done without undue consciousness of the effort involved, but this can only be the case when we have had opportunity of meeting our various needs, and of preserving our confidence in our own capability. Choice of work and efficiency in doing it will be greatly safeguarded if, as a result of good play, we are able to direct our thinking to genuine objective situations, rather than to seemingly objective problems serving as a disguise for more personal preoccupations. Such activity cannot be work of the most effective kind. Further, if our play has been and still is satisfactory, we shall not expect from our work satisfaction of a kind which it cannot give, and consequently shall be relieved of the need to hang disgruntled feeling on work as the nearest peg. Humdrum work will be better tolerated if relieved by good recreation. Satisfactory play, with its social implications, provides us with a sound foundation, and progressive support for every aspect of development. Without it, the child's more formal education will be of little avail in helping him to the harmonizing of his personality.

II. EDUCATIONAL GUIDANCE

By Constance Simmins, M.A., Educational Psychologist, Institute of Medical Psychology

II. EDUCATIONAL GUIDANCE

BY CONSTANCE SIMMINS, M.A., EDUCATIONAL
PSYCHOLOGIST, INSTITUTE OF MEDICAL
PSYCHOLOGY

MANY parents realize to-day the importance of *Vocational* Guidance, of selecting congenial and suitable work for their boys and girls when they leave school. They know that it is not good to force a round peg into a square hole. Vocational misfit means boredom, strain and possible failure. It is not yet sufficiently recognized that an *educational* misfit has even more disastrous consequences. The damage done strikes deeper and the effects may be permanent. Though change of work may be difficult, it is not impossible. But school years cannot be re-lived. If they are misspent, no second chance is given, and the child may enter adult life ill-equipped and maladjusted, a potential misfit in life and work.

By *educational guidance* is meant the selection of a particular type of school or teaching to suit the capacities and needs of a particular child. The choice is made, on the one hand, on a basis of knowledge about the child, his intelligence, his special gifts and his interests, and, on the other hand, on a basis of knowledge about available educational facilities. Before deciding what kind of education is likely to be most suitable for a child two questions must be answered : First, what is this child's mind like, how intelligent is he, does he show any special aptitude, has he any interests that are likely to endure and to be of value to him ? Secondly, what kinds of education are available for this child from the point of view of locality and cost ?

THE CHILD'S MIND

Intelligence

It has been said that " it is a wise parent that knows his own child ", and it is indeed difficult even for the wisest of parents to be sufficiently detached to judge their children fairly and accurately. Parents in the nature of things cannot easily take an unbiased view. There is the very natural desire that one's own child should excel and every goose is a swan. On the other hand, a father who cannot forget his own very mediocre performances at school may find it difficult to acknowledge superior ability in his son. Then, again, some parents have little or no experience of other children and therefore lack standards of comparison. There are families where the first child is very retarded or even mentally defective, but the young parents did not realize that there was anything abnormal about the child's mental development, until the far more rapid development of a second child made them anxious about the older one. Many parents have no conception of their children's ability as compared with other children, until their children have attended school for some time. Then position in school or class may reveal to surprised parents that they have a child exceptionally bright or, it may be, exceptionally dull. But this knowledge is gained too late to help them in their choice of education. Many years may already have been wasted in a school of the wrong type for that particular child.

A teacher is, of course, better able than the parents to assess accurately a child's intelligence. He deals with many children and so has a standard of comparison. He can compare the learning capacity of one child with that of others of his age. But, even so, his judgment is not infallible. Though learning capacity is determined mainly by intelligence, not all children make effective use of their intelligence in school work. They may be distracted or inhibited by emotional disturbances, or they may be handicapped by some undiscovered physical defect or disorder. In such circumstances a bright child may appear, even to the experienced teacher, to be mediocre or even dull, a child of average ability may appear to be almost mentally defective. The teacher's opinion may, therefore, fall wide of the mark. In any case, it may come too late for early guidance in education.

If the opinions of parents and teachers are not reliable or, at best, come too late, we are bound to seek some more exact and more reliable method of discovering the potential capacity of the child. Fortunately for the children of this and of future generations there is a better way. A child's intelligence can be measured by tests. At this point the reader may object that it is unreasonable of psychologists to claim that they can measure intelligence, when they do not seem able to tell us what intelligence is. The psychologist is quite justified in meeting this objection by pointing out that there are in the physical world forces operating which are not yet fully understood, but which can nevertheless be measured. We may not understand the ultimate nature of electricity, but we accept the reading of our metre and pay our bill without objecting that what is not fully comprehended cannot be measured.

Intelligence has been variously described as " adaptability to new situations ", " the power of good responses from the point of view of truth ", " abstract thinking ", " the capacity to profit by experience ", " inborn, all-round mental efficiency " —a complete account of the descriptions and definitions offered by psychologists would only add to our confusion. The truth is that even among psychologists the concept of " intelligence " is vague and evades definition. We shall be on safer ground if we consider what the so-called " intelligence " tests actually measure. They measure " a factor which enters into the measurement of ability of all kinds, and which is throughout constant for any individual, although varying greatly for different individuals ".[1] It is useful and, in the present state of our knowledge, permissible to explain this factor as " mental energy ", which functions primarily and essentially in the educing of relations and correlates, that is, in the bringing to

[1] Spearman, *The Abilities of Man*, 1927, p. 411.

awareness of the relations between things experienced, and in the mental production of ideas required to fit into given relational systems. While the psychologist talks of " educing relations " the man in the street talks of " seeing how things hang together ", of " getting the hang of things ", and means much the same thing. The psychologist " educes correlates " and the man in the street " puts two and two together " and, if he " makes four ", he has produced the idea that necessarily fits into and completes that particular system of relations.

A good intelligence test measures a child's power of eduction, his ability to " get the hang of things ", to " put two and two together ". No one will deny that to be reasonably well endowed with this power is one of the necessary conditions of successful living and to be poorly endowed with it is one of life's greatest handicaps. Each individual is endowed at birth with a certain, definite amount of this mental power or " general ability ", which normally increases during childhood until it reaches its maximum at about the age of sixteen. Individual differences in general ability extend over a very wide range from intellectual genius at one end of the scale to imbecility and idiocy at the other. " Intelligence " Tests show sufficiently accurately for all practical purposes whether a child is of average intelligence or whether, and to what extent, he is above or below the average.

The first tests to establish themselves widely in general use were those devised and standardized by the French psychologist Binet. They have stood the test of time and are to-day more widely used than any other tests for the individual measurement of a child's intelligence. Though they no longer meet the requirements of present-day psychologists, their practical usefulness and general reliability are beyond question. To Binet we owe, also, the ingenious and very valuable device of the "age scale", by which it is possible to calculate the child's *mental age* directly from the test results. His tests are arranged in groups of from four to eight tests, each group being allotted to a year of age, from three years to sixteen.[1] When Binet found during the standardizing of his tests that approximately 60 per cent. of the children of a particular age passed a test successfully, he considered this test suitable for children of that age, neither too difficult nor too easy for them. Four of the tests for eight-year-olds (as they appear in the widely used Stanford Revision of the Binet Tests) [1] are given below as samples :

1. Count backwards from 20 to 0.
   The time allowed is 40 seconds and one error is permitted.
2. What is the thing for you to do :
   a. When you have broken something that belongs to someone else ?
   b. When you are on your way to school and notice that you are in danger of being late ?
   c. If a playmate hits you without meaning to do it ?
   Two out of the three questions must be answered sensibly.

[1] Terman, *The Measurement of Intelligence*, 1919.

3. In what way are wood and coal alike ? An apple and a peach ? Iron and silver ? A ship and a motor-car ?

   Two of the four questions must be answered correctly.

4. The child must be able to give the meaning of 20 words in a given list (gown, orange, tap, bonfire, scorch, straw, etc.).

If an eight-year-old child passes all the tests for his age, but fails to pass any of the slightly more difficult tests for the ninth year, his *mental age* is eight, he has done what most other children of his age do in these tests, it is assumed that he is of *average* intelligence. If he passes tests allotted to ages higher than his own, he is above the average, or advanced in intelligence. If he cannot pass the tests for his age, but succeeds only in passing those for younger children, he is below the average, or retarded in intelligence. His exact mental age can be calculated in years and months. The next step is to find the child's *Intelligence Quotient* by a simple formula : $\dfrac{\text{Mental Age} \times 100}{\text{Actual Age}}$. It is obvious that, if mental age and actual (or chronological) age are the same the I.Q. is 100. An I.Q. of 100, then, indicates average intelligence. The value of the I.Q. lies in the fact that it tends to remain constant. If a child is re-tested after an interval of one, two, or more years his mental age will of course have increased, but the *relation between* his mental age and his actual age remains the same. The child of eight with a mental age of ten will, when ten years old, have a mental age of twelve and a half, and when twelve years old, a mental age of fifteen. The child's I.Q. of 125, that is, the ratio of his mental age to his actual age, remains the same. Because the I.Q. is constant it is possible on the results of an intelligence test given at an early age to foretell what a child's learning capacity will be during school years, and, within wide limits, what types of work will be within his capacity when he leaves school.

The following table quoted by Burt in a report of the Industrial Fatigue Research Board shows the significance of different intelligence quotients for education and work.

Since the first appearance of the Binet Tests an immense number of intelligence tests, both verbal and non-verbal, have been devised. This is not the place to enumerate even the best of them. The reader who is interested in mental testing is referred to two recent publications : *The Testing of Intelligence* (ed. Hamley),[1] and *A Guide to Mental Testing*, by Cattell.[2]

SPECIAL ABILITIES

While educational guidance should not be attempted without knowing how intelligent the child is, there are other factors that should be taken into account, factors which will still further limit the choice of school ; especially for older children. Many children show liking for or facility in music, art, literature, drama, or handicrafts, to mention only a few of the talents and special aptitudes that

[1] *The Testing of Intelligence*, published by Evans Bros., 1936.
[2] *A Guide to Mental Testing*, Cattell, 1936.

TABLE OF EDUCATIONAL AND VOCATIONAL CATEGORIES *

Mental Ratio.	Educational Category.	Per cent. of Children.	Vocational Category.	Per cent. of Adults.
150 +	Scholarships (Univ. hons.)	0·2	Highest prof. administrative	0·1
130/150	Scholarships (Secondary)	2	Lower prof. and tech.	3
115/130	Central and Higher Elem.	10	Clerical and highly skilled	12
100/115	Ordinary Elem.	38	Skilled and ordinary commercial	26
85/100	Ordinary Elem.	38	Semi-skilled and poorest commercial	33
70/85	Dull and backward classes	10	Unskilled and coarse manual labour	19
50/70	Special and M.D. schools	1·5	Casual labour	7
50 −	Ineducable	0·2	Institutional (Imbeciles and Idiots)	0·2

* *N.B.*—This table, quoted with the kind permission of Professor Burt, was compiled some years ago. At the present time the percentage of elementary school-children proceeding to Central and Secondary Schools is considerably higher. In the London area the lower limit of I.Q. for Central School education is now approximately 112 and that for Secondary School education approximately 127. In other parts of the country the standards show wide variations.

a child may possess over and above his intelligence or general ability. While it would be mistaken to sacrifice a broad general education to the development of a talent or aptitude, however great, it would be equally mistaken to set the child in a school environment which allowed no scope for the exercise and development of his talent. A boy with a scientific turn of mind would, for example, be cramped and thwarted in a school without a laboratory.

Special aptitudes may be dormant during early childhood. Some cannot appear until a certain stage of neurological development has been reached. Some only come to light in response to an appropriate stimulus. Special talents demand as a rule some special kind of material or experience to draw them forth and to nourish them. If the child's environment is lacking in the appropriate elements, potential talent may be dormant and undiscovered. Though some special aptitudes, music, for example, are undoubtedly inborn, others are rather of the nature of " skills ", acquired through opportunity, interest and practice.

Some aptitudes, whether inborn or acquired, can be measured, but the tests available are less reliable than those which measure " intelligence ". Amongst the more satisfactory and promising of the tests of special aptitude are Seashore's Musical Talent Test, the Meier-Seashore Art Judgment Test and Cox's Test of Mechanical Aptitude.[1] What is more important than any attempt to measure special abilities is the provision from the earliest years of a soil of rich and varied opportunity, where a child's talent will spring up and grow, whatever that talent may be.

[1] For detailed information about these and other tests of special aptitudes see Cattell, *A Guide to Mental Testing*, 1936.

EDUCATIONAL DISABILITIES

When are we justified in saying that a child suffers from a " disability " ?   Certainly not when he happens to be lacking in some special talent, possessed only by a minority.   The term " disability " should be reserved for inability to do some one kind of thing that most other children of his age can do.   Thus it is permissible to speak of a disability in reading, writing, spelling, arithmetic or handwork.   It is not permissible to speak of a disability in music, art or dramatic work.   A disability may be caused by some inherent weakness, but in most cases it is due to the inhibiting effect of unfavourable experiences, past or present.

The most common inherent weaknesses or defects, which may handicap a child in learning one or more of the school subjects, are defective sight, deafness, and weakness in visual or auditory memory.   If defective vision is discovered and corrected by glasses before the child goes to school no harm is done.   A slight defect of hearing may escape detection and the child may pass through school without anyone discovering that he hears less clearly than the other children.   If he does not hear speech-sounds clearly, his own speech will be indistinct and his spelling poor.   A seat in the front row of the class might have saved him from " disabilities " in speech and spelling.   Weak visual or auditory memory is not necessarily a serious handicap, though they may result in " disability " or backwardness in reading, spelling or arithmetic, if the child is taught by rigid and unsuitable methods.   There are more ways than one of teaching each of the fundamental school subjects. The child whose visual memory is weak will learn best by using ears, hands and speech; the child with poor auditory memory will learn best by using eyes, hands and speech. Teaching methods should be elastic and readily adjustable to the needs of the individual child. A twelve-year-old girl was referred to an educational psychologist on account of her inability to spell correctly. She was of average intelligence and her attendance at school had been regular. She had musical ability and a fine ear not only for musical sounds, but also for speech-sounds. She spelt phonetically and therefore inaccurately. She was found to be extremely weak in visual memory. She could not retain the " look " of a word, however often she saw it or however carefully she attended to it. Under a specially devised system of instruction, which made considerable demands on her auditory memory, but none on her visual memory, her spelling steadily improved. Children with weak auditory memory often find difficulty in learning the multiplication tables by heart. They can, however, learn and remember them by seeing, writing and understanding them.

More frequent and more serious causes of disability or backwardness in a school subject are rooted in feeling and emotion. If the first lessons in reading, for example, are not pleasant and interesting to the child, a feeling of " not liking " attaches itself to the reading lesson and the child will not, and indeed cannot attend.

An eight-year-old boy was sent to an educational psychologist for coaching in reading, in which he was very backward. At the first lesson attractive reading material was set out, but his response to it was : " I don't like reading." However, a friendly contact was established and a little work done, half-heartedly and because he did not like to risk " naughtiness " with a stranger. On the second occasion different and even more attractive material was displayed, but this time his reaction was an outburst of : " I hate the very sight of this." But more work was done and with a better will than on the first occasion. He seemed to be discovering that the teacher was not going to be cross or impatient, that he was quite able to do what he was asked to do and that the whole business was more like a game than a lesson. From that time onwards there was no further difficulty. The unpleasant associations had been ousted by pleasant ones. It would have been far more difficult to help this boy a year or two later, for by that time the situation would have become more complex. Feelings of discouragement, fright and inferiority would have been added to the initial feeling of " not liking ". The result is an unhappy state of conflict, which makes learning difficult if not impossible. Occasionally, a child will find his own solution of the conflict by accepting the situation with placidity : " Reading is one of the things I can't do." It may even happen that a child has a strong incentive *not* to learn to read. A boy of nine had not mastered even the elements of reading. In the course of conversation with him it appeared that neither his father nor his grandfather had been able to read. Both had been professional football players and it was the boy's ambition to follow in their footsteps, but in his experience a good football player did not read, therefore he was not going to run the risk of allowing reading to spoil his chances on the football field.

If a child, at any stage in his school career, falls behind through a spell of illness or for any other reason, he finds himself handicapped, not only by lack of knowledge, but also by feelings of bewilderment, discouragement and self-mistrust. The result may be a wholehearted dislike of school, and in some cases physical illness, truancy or a definite refusal to go to school at all. A little girl greatly enjoyed her first year in the Infant School, then influenza followed by bronchitis kept her away for several weeks. Meanwhile her class had progressed in reading and number work, and on her return she felt herself to be the dunce of the class. Her mother reported that the child did not seem to like school now and that she was not making progress. Fortunately this child was in a small class under a teacher who soon realized what was amiss. The child was given individual attention, with the result that the lost ground was soon regained. The child once more enjoyed school and made good progress.

With older children the subject most sensitive to absence is mathematics. If the explanation of a new rule is missed, then, unless someone takes the trouble to explain the rule and give some practice in its application, there will be bewilderment and inaccuracy, which will prevent further progress. An intelligent boy of fifteen was regarded as hopeless in Algebra. Individual coaching revealed that he had never mastered the way to deal with plus and minus signs in subtracting and multiplying. Explanation and the working of examples under supervision soon cleared up the difficulty and he began to gain high marks in this subject at school. Most children need expert and sympathetic guiding through the dangerous period that follows a spell of absence. Though some children by means of their good intelligence combined with a determination to succeed will regain the lost ground by questioning teachers, parents or schoolfellows, or by reference to text-books, there is no doubt that the majority need some special help and encouragement, if harmful consequences are to be avoided.

Tests have been devised both to measure the degree of a child's backwardness in reading, spelling, English and arithmetic and also to show where is the gap in his knowledge or the weakness in his learning ability. Full accounts of such tests and their uses will be found in *Mental and Scholastic Tests*, by Burt, and in *The Testing of Intelligence*, edited by Hamley. It is not, however, necessary to apply such tests in every case of backwardness. One of the best ways of discovering the causes of backwardness and the means of remedying it is to allow an educational psychologist or a skilful and sympathetic teacher to give the child individual teaching of an experimental kind. Burt defines the experimental teaching of a backward child in this way :

It consists of individual instruction carried out by constantly varied devices and by widely diversified methods ; but it is accompanied always by a close observation of the child's spontaneous method of attack, and by a detailed study of the ways which the child can, does, and will by preference, follow and adopt in learning a given piece of work ; and it is to be succeeded always by an intensive training in the most defective operations by means of the least defective mental channels.[1]

CHILDREN'S INTERESTS

Should we allow a child's interests to affect our choice of school ? To every child at every age there are certain kinds of objects or certain activities which matter to him, which are of great importance to him and absorb much of his thought and energy. Many of these interests are evanescent, belonging to a particular phase of his development and yielding in due course to other interests, which oust the earlier ones. A small boy may be absorbed in the activities of a bus conductor for weeks or months at a time, but no parent would be misguided enough to take this as an indication of his future career and plan his education in accordance with it.

Even where a child shows interests of more enduring quality caution should be exercised, before assuming that the child's true " bent " lies in this direction. In a narrow, dull environment the child's energies will find an outlet where they can and not where they would if the environment were richer in opportunity. In an old-fashioned boarding school, where the lessons were exceedingly dreary, a girl's main interests were needlework, painting, swimming and gymnastics. On removal to a school where there was good teaching in all subjects the earlier interests swiftly subsided, to be

[1] Burt, *Mental and Scholastic Tests*, 1927, p. 268.

replaced by intellectual interests which lasted into adult life and determined her subsequent career.

Then, again, a child's interests may be determined and maintained by his parents, who may set a high value on some one kind of performance. In an unmusical family mediocre aptitude for piano playing may be rated far too high. The child's interest in the piano may be more a form of exhibitionism than a sign of true talent. The undue encouragement by ambitious parents of an aptitude, that is in fact mediocre, may lead to bitter disillusionment in later years.

In a minority of cases an interest may be pathological in origin and a symptom of psychological disorder. Only after psychological treatment will the child be able to develop interests that are normal. An adolescent girl of abnormal emotional development was interested in old men with beards, counting the number seen each day, as a child might count his marbles or cigarette cards.

If a child's interests may be evanescent, spurious or even pathological, should a regard for his interests play any part in our attempt to guide him educationally? Definitely yes! For free and full development it is of the greatest importance that his Kindergarten and his junior or preparatory school should offer wide and varied opportunities to attract and develop interests suitable to his age, thus making good environmental deficiencies of his pre-school days and allowing full scope for any interests which he may already possess. When the time comes to pass into a senior department or a public school the boy or girl may have already developed

some interest of real value, which will be an enduring source of pleasure and satisfaction to him.
Such interests should be taken seriously into account
in choosing the school in which he will probably
spend the remaining years of his school life. Most
schools for boys and girls over fourteen years of age
plan their curriculum to meet the requirements of
the General Schools Examination and there may be
little time or opportunity for activities outside the
scope of the examination, though practically all
schools encourage sport. A boy or girl of good
ability, sociable and interested in games is likely to
progress well and happily in any good school,
though even with these fortunate ones it is wise to
take into account any special ability or interest they
may have and to choose a school that allows scope
for its development. Not all good schools encourage musical or dramatic talent. Some have no
workshop or laboratory. Many girls' schools still
have no domestic science department and no teaching of handicrafts. If it is at all possible, the school
chosen should have a department that makes provision for the child's particular interest or aptitude,
besides providing a sound all-round education fitted
to his intellectual capacity.

EDUCATIONAL OPPORTUNITY

Each year the chances of finding the kind of
education to meet the needs of the individual child
increase. Well-equipped Nursery Schools, classes
for carpentry, metal-work, domestic science, music
and art in the Elementary Schools, free places in
Trade, Technical, Central and Secondary Schools,

offer elementary school-children in many of our larger towns a rich and varied educational environment, in which they have a reasonably good opportunity of developing, in accordance with their intellectual capacity, their interests and their special aptitudes. Though many districts, particularly agricultural areas, are still far behind in the provision of a sufficiently varied educational service, the education authorities are working slowly but surely towards an ideal, which aims at providing every child in the elementary schools with the kind of education that he needs.

The educational authorities are, however, not only responsible for the provision of adequate educational opportunities but also for the guiding of each individual child into the path where his special needs will be met and his special gifts developed. Much of this guidance occurs automatically within the educational framework provided. In the larger schools the child of superior intellectual capacity will find himself moving up the school in the divisions for brighter children, while the child of average ability will pass through the school in divisions, where a less exacting standard will be required of him. In many schools there is also a " track " laid down for dull children, where they are taught at a slower pace and by methods specially adapted to their more limited intelligence, and where more time is devoted to development along practical lines. One of the outstanding needs of the present time is a great increase in the number of such classes for dull children and in the facilities for giving special training to carefully selected teachers for these classes. The dull child, unless suitably taught by specially adapted methods, may easily fail to learn up to his capacity. The methods of teaching suitable to children of average ability are not simple and concrete enough for him to grasp and the rate of progress is too fast for him. At the end of his school years he may be illiterate and his mind may be permanently damaged by an unhappy and unprofitable school life. Instead of becoming a social asset, well able to earn his living in unskilled manual work, he becomes a social burden, unemployable, ill-adapted, neurotic and possibly criminal. The expert and sympathetic education of the less intelligent children of the country would go a long way towards solving the social problems of unemployability, crime and mental breakdown.

Some of the more progressive education authorities take very seriously their responsibility for guiding each child into the path where his needs will be most adequately met. They arrange for the testing of each child's intelligence at about the age of eight years, with the aim that every child, without unnecessary and harmful delay, shall be placed in the class or school where he will be able to learn according to his capacity. A few education authorities enhance the value of the intelligence test results by giving educational tests as well to discover which children are already backward for their capacity. Where there is a disparity between the child's intelligence and his educational achievements, the causes of this disparity may then be investigated and every effort made to help the child towards normal progress. These efforts may take the form of a change of school or class, of special individual teaching for a time, or expert advice given by a psychologist, home visits by a specially trained social worker or treatment at a Child Guidance Clinic, if one is available.

What of the non-elementary school-children, children whose parents pay fees for their education? For these the provision of educational opportunities depends largely upon private enterprise. Educational guidance lies in the first instance with the parents. At a later stage, advice may be offered by the head-master or head-mistress of the child's school. The elementary school-child attends as a matter of course one of the elementary schools near his home. The fee-paying pupil goes to a school chosen by his parents. The parents may be guided solely by expedience, selecting the nearest day-school that suits their purse. Or family tradition may be the determining factor and the child is sent to the school where his father or elder brothers were educated. Sometimes ambition settles the choice. The boy must go to one of the great public schools and after that to Oxford or Cambridge. Where expediency, family tradition or parental ambition determine the choice of school, there is a complete ignoring of the child himself, his capacities and his special needs. Far too much is left to chance. The school thus selected may by good luck suit the child. On the other hand it may totally fail to provide either the kind of teaching or the kind of environment that would call forth and develop the child's capacities and interests. It may, in consequence, have a definitely repressive and crippling effect upon him, so that he leaves school ill-adjusted to life instead of educated for life.

The child who has been set upon the wrong educational road is fortunate if, within the first year or two, disastrous consequences in the shape of bad school reports, abnormal behaviour or ill-health drive the parents to seek expert advice and a change of school is made in time to avoid permanent ill-effects. Some parents take the matter into their own hands and send the unfortunate child to a " crammers ", sacrificing him to their own ambitions. The boy must at all costs enter a Public School. Such boys spend childhood and adolescence in an atmosphere of failure and criticism. They never know the satisfaction either of successful achievement or of parental approval. They come to regard themselves as failures, and failures they become.

There are children whose education has been wrong from the outset. In the early years there may have been a governess, or a succession of governesses, chosen in ignorance of the kind of training and personality desirable in a teacher of young children. Or the child may have been sent to the kind of school, which unhappily still exists as a direct descendant of the old " dame schools ", where all the school hours are spent in learning reading, writing, spelling and arithmetic. With this narrow curriculum there goes hand-in-hand an old-fashioned and rigid method of teaching. The child may well dislike and resent the tedious hours and waste his time in naughtiness or day-dreaming. With the first years wasted he will then go to a preparatory school without the necessary groundwork and without the happy adjustment to school life that would have resulted from beginning in a good Kindergarten or with a small group of children under a sympathetic and well-trained governess. At the preparatory school the unfortunate child makes a bad start. He does not know as much as the other new-comers, he is discouraged and discomfited, he dislikes the school. He goes home at the end of term with a bad report. And so the dreary tale goes on, with disapproval, scolding, punishment even, all along the line. There is no real happiness for him, no security, no chance of developing self-confidence either at home or at school. The parents are disappointed, bewildered and resentful. The child is fast becoming a social problem as well as an educational one.

Such tragedies can be avoided. Above all things let the child-begin well. Let his early education be entrusted to people who understand the art of making learning as pleasant and absorbing to the child as his play, and who will know how to provide him with all the materials and experiences that he needs for full and happy development. When he passes out of the Kindergarten stage he should attend a school with a definitely happy atmosphere and a curriculum wide enough to include music, art and a number of practical activities in addition to the usual lessons and organized games. It is at the same time of the greatest importance that the school selected should not give him occasion to feel either intellectually inferior or intellectually starved. If he is not of good intelligence schools that set store by academic success should be avoided.

When he is ready to enter upon the final years of school life, a school should be chosen where, again, he will not be an intellectual misfit and where opportunity is offered for the encouragement and development of any special aptitudes or enduring interests that may by this time have made their appearance.

There will always be some exceptional children who remain " problem " children, unable to respond satisfactorily even to the most favourable educational environment. These are children handicapped either by some serious inherent weakness, or by some deep-seated emotional disturbance having its origin in infantile experiences or in disharmonious or peculiar circumstances in the home. These special cases need special treatment by a child psychiatrist before they can make a normal adjustment to school life.

Before effective educational guidance can be given to every child in the country much remains to be done. We need, in the first place, a great increase in the number of certain types of schools and classes. We need more nursery schools, more classes for practical work of varied kinds and more special classes and schools providing suitable and expert teaching for the less intelligent children. The application of intelligence tests and educational tests at about eight years of age would be a safeguard against educational misplacement and consequent psychological harm. Many more psychological advisers should be appointed and many more Child Guidance Clinics opened to bring expert advice within the reach of all. Most important of all is the need for wider appreciation by parents and teachers of the harmful consequences of an unsuitable education.

III. THE ADOLESCENT GIRL

By Laura Hutton, B.A., M.R.C.S., L.R.C.P.,
Physician, Tavistock Clinic (Institute of
Medical Psychology)

III. THE ADOLESCENT GIRL

BY LAURA HUTTON, B.A., M.R.C.S., L.R.C.P.,
PHYSICIAN, TAVISTOCK CLINIC (INSTITUTE OF
MEDICAL PSYCHOLOGY)

THOSE of us who have lived with growing children, and have been observant—perhaps school-mistresses, with their daily contact with numbers of girls, have the best opportunity for such observations—must have noted a twice-recurring, indefinable change come over girls in the course of their growth. There comes a day when one notes on the face of the little girl of the third or fourth form (or first or second year, in the newer terminology), whom one has hitherto classed among " the little ones ", a peculiar change—indefinable yet definite—a change which records itself in one's observing mind as : " This is a young girl—this is no longer a child." One gets used to that somehow oddly-lengthened face, with its deepened significance that distinguishes it from the rounded and unaware face of the child of yesterday ; and one watches a rapidly growing and developing person, now all angles, now all bulges, full of awkwardnesses, moods and withdrawals, and often very plain of countenance. And then another day comes when one is startled by seeing a suddenly (it appears) beautiful creature before one—poised, self-confident and expectant. And again one's observing mind records : " This is no longer a young girl, this is a young woman."

I take as adolescence the period between these two definite, observable, but undefinable changes in the outward appearance of girls, i.e. the period between roughly twelve and eighteen or nineteen.

PHYSICAL CHANGES OF ADOLESCENCE

We will deal first with the physical aspects of adolescence.

The onset of menstruation is the outstanding physical event of adolescence in girls, but this event only marks a stage in a far-reaching physical development and reorganization. The secondary sexual characteristics begin to manifest themselves usually at least a year, sometimes considerably longer, before the onset of menstruation. The development of the breasts, preceded sometimes by many months of tenderness, may be quite far advanced, and the pubic hair usually appears a year before the first period. These things being so, there is ample opportunity for the girl to be instructed about the period before its first appearance, and no excuse for letting her be taken by surprise and perhaps alarmed. But instruction, certainly much more regularly given now than hitherto, must be of the right kind. The sentimental vagueness, for example, of the little booklets contained in packets of sanitary towels is *not* a model for such instruction! Such vagueness can do no more than irritate and perplex an intelligent girl, and perhaps even alarm. Anything that suggests the period as a monthly handicap, a being *unwell*, is to be avoided, as also suggestions of its being a " cleansing of the system ". Both these suggestions are false in fact, and bad in effect, making the girl associate the mark of her development to maturity with inferiority and disgust.

The truth is, on the contrary, good to hear. The period is the sign that her ovaries are now capable of producing ripe seeds, and her womb accordingly sets going its cycle of a monthly preparation for the receiving of a seed, which, if fertilized, will develop from an embryo to a baby ready to be born. For a time no fertilization of the seed will take place, for that is the part her husband in the future has to fulfil ; but that does not prevent the monthly cycle from taking place. It is a bodily rhythm which will be maintained until her ovaries have no more seeds to ripen, when she is round about fifty.

THE PSYCHOLOGICAL SIGNIFICANCE OF MENSTRUATION

There is nothing horrifying or disgusting about this, and the girl who has learned any botany will understand what fertilization means and be ready for fuller information as to the husband's part. But there is no need to force this on her, if she seems unwilling to hear it. It is a problem to which we will return later.

There is a special reason why it is important that instructions about the period should be given in a way calculated to raise a girl's sense of her significance as a woman and a potential mother.

73

It is connected with early experiences and fantasies which occur in the lives of many small girls. The little girl, when first she sees a baby boy, is struck by the fact that his body has something which hers lacks. Many little girls point this out immediately; others, in whom repression of the earliest instinctual impulses has already been extreme (and it is astonishing how early such repression can take place in a sensitive child with an anxious or exacting mother), may appear not to notice anything, and yet be even more profoundly affected. Unless this situation—the first realization of the difference between boys and girls—is handled with understanding and tact, the little girl may grow up with an unconscious (i.e. repressed and forgotten) fantasy that she has been deprived of this organ, that it has been cut off by some grown-up. She bitterly resents the loss, for it is an organ which obviously offers many advantages; for instance, the pleasure of holding it and seeing its power to eject a stream. We would need to be very blind not to notice how keen this pleasure is to small boys, and some of us may have had experience of little girls who have literally tried to imitate their brothers in this— only to be met with ignominious disappointment. This fantasy—that a part of herself has been cut off—may have a profound influence on the psychological development of a little girl, making her consciously or unconsciously long to be a boy, and hate to admit that she is a girl. To such a girl the appearance of her first period may be a very critical experience. To her unconscious mind it may confirm the fantasy of being injured, wounded, long ago, and thus stir up a secret fear and revolt beyond anything she can understand. To her *un-conscious* mind, I repeat ; for there is no question of such a fantasy as I have described being consciously in the thoughts of a girl of twelve or fourteen. But modern psychology has taught us one thing of paramount importance in the understanding of emotional disturbances, and that is that such disturbances are as frequently the result of unconscious thoughts, fears and impulses as they are of conscious mental activity. To the girl's *conscious* mind the period is a declaration of her femininity. To both these experiences, the conscious as well as the unconscious, she may react with a violent protest, rejecting her womanhood and resenting its manifestation. She may consciously wish to be a boy ; many girls do feel, not always without reason, that boys and men have a better time than girls and women. The appearance of the period puts the prospect before her of inevitable womanhood, and there is a good deal to be renounced before this can be accepted. In her unconscious mind things are even worse, for here the period seems, as we have suggested, to be a confirmation of her belief that she has been injured —probably as a punishment for some infantile activity, such as "playing with herself" (masturbation).

To many people this may seem a far-fetched account of a girl's possible emotional reaction to her first period. Needless to say, I am not suggesting that all girls, or even the majority, react in this way. But the analysis of adults has shown that to quite a number of girls, the onset of menstruation does represent an upsetting experience in the way I have described. Such girls are likely to suffer from intractable dysmenorrhœa (pain and sickness at the time of the period), as each month they unconsciously renew their protest at this confirmation of their worst fears and denial of their dearest wish. And later, in marriage, they will probably be unhappy or dissatisfied in their sexual life with their husbands. I must repeat, to avoid misunderstanding, that most of the protest I have described is unconscious : only in an occasional case will there be a conscious revolt against menstruation, because it stands for womanhood in a girl who wants to be a boy. But as I have already indicated, modern psychology has taught us how small in comparison with the active totality of our minds is the conscious part of it, and how profoundly our behaviour and even our physical experiences are determined by motives, wishes and fears that never reach consciousness.

In view of all this, then, we see how important it is that this opportunity of the onset of menstruation (or rather the indications that point to it) should be taken to help growing girls to overcome any resentment, conscious or unconscious, against their girlhood, and to accept their womanhood as something valuable and significant, offering joys and satisfactions in the future. If menstruation is felt as a handicap or looked upon as a " cleansing " (implying uncleanness), it means that a valuable opportunity has been lost in the education of the adolescent girl for womanhood and motherhood.

Menstruation should be looked upon, and all our instructions should reveal it, as evidence of the vital functioning of a body capable of motherhood.

PUBERTY AND THE ENDOCRINE BALANCE

Just as the cessation of the periods is only one event in the protracted readjustment of the second change of life, the climacteric, so, as has been suggested, is the onset of menstruation one event in the first " change of life "—adolescence. The change is marked by a rearrangement of the endocrine balance of the body, which is demanded when the ovaries begin to form seed follicles and discharge ripe ova, and the thymus gland disappears. And just as at the climacteric the readjustment of the gland balance is marked by transient symptoms of maladjustment, e.g. the hot flushes, so in adolescence there may be symptoms of a similar maladjustment. Skeletal growth may be sudden and excessive; there may be phases of lethargy or excessive nervousness, and a liability to blush without much cause. It is impossible to distinguish or to know at all, sometimes, how much of these evidences of maladjustment are physiological and how much emotional in origin; both factors are usually present. But the tendency has perhaps been to label all the fluctuations and awkwardnesses of the adolescent as signs of emotional instability, and to overlook the part which a physiological gland imbalance is playing. There is at the present time not enough definite knowledge available to enable doctors to prescribe confidently for such imbalance, even when it is suspected as a factor in a given

77

case of " adolescent instability ", but it is nevertheless worth while to take some trouble to estimate
this factor, since doing so will modify our psychological handling of the problems presented, and
perhaps enable us in some cases to take a less
serious view of them, as ominous for the girl's
future.

THE DEVELOPING LOVE-LIFE OF THE ADOLESCENT GIRL

To turn to the psychological problems of the
adolescent girl : the first one to strike the psychologist, though perhaps not always the parent, is that
of her developing love-life.

I have here suggested an opposition between
the point of view of the psychologist and that of
the parent, an antagonism which is too often suspected, and does something to stultify the efforts
of the psychologist to be helpful. So before going
further, let me try to remove any sense of such
antagonism by going a little deeper into the question. One must remember that the psychologist,
when presented with an adolescent girl, sees her
primarily as an adolescent girl—someone, that is
to say, who is in a transitional phase, *en route* to
adulthood. He by no means overlooks the childhood out of which she is evolving, but to him the
important point is that she is growing up, going
forward ; and his first thought is of the potential
adult before him. The parent—let us say mother,
as it is usually the mother with whom one has to
deal—on the other hand, has been in close touch
with the child from infancy. Hers is a more day-

by-day awareness, in which changes come almost imperceptibly, and it is much easier for her to see in the adolescent girl someone who, as one may put it, has outgrown her socks than as someone who is nearly ready for a latchkey. Indeed, many parents find it very difficult to recognize that the socks *are* outgrown, and that it is not mere tiresomeness that has spoiled their fit. Yet, as we see, their point of view is not really antagonistic to that of the psychologist, but is the natural result of past experience. What the psychologist, unhampered by this past, does spontaneously—i.e. see in the adolescent the nearly adult person—most parents have to make an effort to do; for to them their daughter is first and foremost their " little girl ", the little girl she has been from nursery days.

Such a parent as I have described may be reluctant to admit the thought of a developing love-life in her adolescent daughter. Yet it is clear that, as on the physical side the development of sexual maturity is the outstanding event of adolescence, so on the psychological side the development of the capacity to form a full and normal love relationship with a member of the opposite sex is the outstanding psychological (emotional) experience.

Girls develop at very different rates in this respect, just as their sexual endowment and rate of development vary within wide limits. Some girls are looking for " boy friends " at thirteen or fourteen, others are regarding all such interest as " silly " when they go up to College at eighteen or nineteen. The tendency, unfortunately, among school-mistresses and parents is to regard the former with disapproval and anxiety, and the latter with approval and satisfaction. Whereas the chances are that the more seriously maladjusted young people will be found in this second group of " good, sensible girls ", as we shall see later. How hard it is for even the most enlightened people to escape from the tendency to find reassurance in what is often simply evidence of delayed development, was brought home to me recently when I was discussing this very problem of the adolescent girl with an exceedingly able, broadminded and understanding head-mistress. When telling me of a return visit to her school of an old pupil she described how she suggested to the girl, who evidently arrived in full adult war-paint, that she might have a wash before they had their talk; and she told me with every evidence of satisfaction that the girl reappeared in her old school tunic and said "Now I'm more myself, and we can talk better". Even to the best of head-mistresses the girl seemed a better and more satisfactory person *after she had taken a step backwards towards her childhood.* It is extraordinarily deep-seated, this reluctance to see the young, with whom we have been in long and close contact, grow up.

THE PSYCHOLOGY OF THE GIRL BABY

To get a clearer understanding of what happens, what may happen, and what may go wrong, during the evolving of the adolescent girl's love-life, we must take a look backward at her earliest psychological development in babyhood. To both girl babies and boy babies, the mother is the first

" love object "—the first person with whom personal contact is made. The first struggle in birth was with the mother, who thrust the child out of her womb into a world of entirely new sensations ; and though there can be no actual awareness in the child's mind of another person's part in this experience, yet it has been suggested that in this earliest of all psychical experiences begins the conflict between emotions which will later develop into that between love and hate. This experience of conflict—ambivalent feeling—as it is called by psychologists, is renewed in the experience of hunger and the stilling of hunger at the breast ; mother gives, *is*, to the tiny baby, the breast which soothes and is the chief source of comfort and pleasure in its life ; but mother also withholds the breast and the baby's discomfort of hunger is expressed in cries which gradually become those of a desperate rage if its need is not supplied. Here is the dawning of the first personal relationship, out of which ultimately all personal and social relationships develop. It is with the mother, and, as we see, includes feelings not only of love (of the childish craving kind) but also of rage or hate.

A further factor in this first personal relationship with the mother comes into play in connection with all the management of the baby's toilet. Here again is ample scope for feelings of pleasure in mother's caresses and play, and gentle handling of the infant's body ; and for feelings of irritation, resentment and rage, in the demands she makes in connection with training in cleanliness, and in bringing to an end pleasurable experiences. In this last connection, an elaboration of the primitive emotions of pleasure, love and rage arises in the realization by the baby of a demand made by the mother on itself to do something, to be something, which will please her; and the converse of this is the baby's first realization of how it can displease her, and forfeit (so it seems) her love. Here, then, in the first primitive contacts of mother and baby over food and toilet are found the deepest roots of our capacity for personal and social relationships.

As I have suggested, both baby boys and baby girls begin their personal life in the same way, learning (ideally) to establish a happy relationship with the mother, who is the object of their earliest feelings of love. But their future destinies in the field of personal relationships are different. The capacity for personal relationships may be said to be fully evolved when it becomes possible for the individual to take a mate of the opposite sex, to live in physical and mental harmony with him or her, with mutual consideration and enrichment, and to take on the responsibility of producing and rearing children. (May I remind readers here that I am talking now of the development of intimate personal relationships, not of the establishment of social contacts in general—a wider problem—hence the narrowing down of my reference to family relationships.) From the mother-child relationship to this complete and intimate personal relationship with mate is a long journey, and it seems to be longer and more tortuous for girls than for boys. One reason may be that the girl has to change the

sex of her love object. Her first love is a member
of her own sex, but she has to reach a point in her
emotional development where she can renounce
her first love and accept a mate of the opposite
sex; while the boy on the other hand chooses his
mate in the image of his first love. Whatever the
crux of the problem is, it certainly seems clear from
the deep analysis of adults—and Freud himself was
the first to point it out—that women accomplish
some peculiarly " inexorable repression " in infancy
and early childhood; and this fact points by infer-
ence to peculiarly intense emotional conflicts concerning the earliest relationship with the mother;
for it is the intolerably painful which is repressed.
With the father's entrance on the scene—towards
the end of the first year (he can hardly be said to
play as a rule any important psychological rôle in
the child's life before this age)—the little girl's
emotional development gets a fresh stimulus,
namely, towards the establishing of a happy relationship with a member of the opposite sex. But
the period of intense emotional development, involving all the psychic mechanisms of repression,
projection, displacement, compensation and over-
reaction, about which deep psychology teaches us,
is now in full swing, and a great deal of repression
of infantile instinctual impulses and rage will, in
fact, already have been unconsciously carried out.
On the top of all this the little girl now becomes
involved in an intense conflict (of the nature of
which she is quite unaware), between her instinctive attraction to her father, and her profound
dependence on her mother, the mother who has

LAURA HUTTON

nevertheless been at times her apparently cruel frustrator, and is now felt to be her rival in the father's affections. It is impossible to begin to do justice to the " triangle drama " of the small girl, which now plays itself out, as disclosed in the deep analysis of adults and in the play-analysis of little girls. Beside it any adult drama grows pale ; but if we are to appreciate the emotional stresses of the adolescent girl in the maturing of her love-life, we do need to have some appreciation of the welter of repressed conflicts upon which even the most normal girl's emotional development is founded. There is no memory of this drama, of course, for most of it has been, to the child, beyond the power of expression, if not unconscious, and repression of the impulses and anxieties involved has also been an unconscious process.

This second phase of intense psychological development subsides at about the age of five to six, to be to some extent reawakened in adolescence, as we see later.

The girl's task in growing up being thus such an onerous one, from the psychologist's point of view, it follows that any evidence of attraction, and attractiveness, to members of the opposite sex should be welcomed, not recognized with the alarm and misgiving expressed on this subject by only too many parents. Guidance and instruction she may need, but discouragement never.

The attraction and attractiveness is an evidence of dawning psycho-sexual *maturity*, and a girl who manifests these signs should therefore be treated with all the respect and reserve with which one would treat a friend. (This is a point which will perhaps be emphasized to the point of irritation in my readers, yet I feel it cannot be made too often.) In this particular situation the practical points that come to mind are questions of meetings and correspondence with " boy friends ". Nothing is more disastrous to the relationship between a girl and her parents at this time than an intrusive and anxious probing into her friendships. Such anxious probing usually arises out of the intense fear of sex that is harboured, even in these days, by the majority of parents. This fear, felt as an urge to shield their children from any sexual experience, combines with the lack of observation regarding their children's development already referred to, to raise a formidable barrier between parents, especially the mother, and the adolescent daughter. Intrusive probing results inevitably in increasing secretiveness on the part of the daughter, and this intensifies the parents' anxiety, driving them to actions still more offensive to the girl, such as demanding to see letters or even opening them; and thus a vicious circle of ever-widening alienation is formed. The girl for whose well-being the parents are so concerned is removed ever further and further from their reach, in her sense of resentment and outrage, and all this happens at a time when probably she is actually feeling quite uncertain of herself and is in real need of help and guidance. One of the most sophisticated, and by parental standards, " stiff-necked " adolescent girls I have ever known once suddenly said to me : " I'm nothing but a kid inside, really." This girl's mother in an interview with me had said the same about her daughter, only her words were: " B. is such a child really, *I know her so well.*" But between this mother and daughter there is nothing left of confidence, scarcely anything of friendliness. Is not this due to what is involved in the fact that the mother felt she stated the whole truth in this view of her child, while B. was, *by virtue of her growing maturity,* enabled to recognize and admit her immaturity? If this is so, then it suggests that it is only as we appreciate the grown-upness of the adolescent that we shall be able to maintain a helpful (*unexpressed*) contact with the un-grown-up part, the " kid " who is still sometimes in great bewilderment.

But parents must not be too discouraged if in spite of all their sympathy and comprehension their adolescent children seem to look elsewhere for help and guidance in connection with the problems of their developing psycho-sexual life. One must remember that adult sexuality has its roots in babyhood, and in babyhood its beginnings are inextricably involved in the daily experiences connected with toilet and cleanliness-training. These experiences again are equally inextricably bound up with conflict, feelings of being " good " or being " naughty ", in relation to the mother. Hence the dawning experiences of adult sexuality, the first stirrings of sexual feeling in friendship are, for the child, often quite unconsciously related to these difficulties and struggles of babyhood, and to a sense of the mother's censorship. The mother, therefore, is sometimes the last person with whom her adolescent daughter will discuss such feelings or the problems and questions which arise in her mind as a result of them. Still more certainly will this be the case if the mother's own attitude to sexuality is one of anxiety and repudiation, if she herself is frigid in her sexual life; but it may happen even when all is well with the mother in this respect—just because of that early, inevitable relationship between herself and the baby girl. If this is so, then the mother's task, no easy one, is to set aside all jealousy, and to further any attempts of her daughter to find help and guidance elsewhere. One mother complained that her daughter took all her problems to her father instead of to herself. But, how excellent! The danger of mother-fixation in a girl is a much more serious one than that of father-fixation, as we shall see; just because mother-fixation is rooted at the more primitive level of development.

In adolescence, according to Dr. Ernest Jones,[1] there is a recapitulation of the emotional development of the first five years, especially in regard to what is known as the Œdipus Complex—the attraction of the child to the parent of opposite sex, and hostility to that of the same sex, as rival. That something like this does happen is borne out by observation of adolescent girls, who do characteristically tend to a greater demonstrativeness towards the father at the age of about twelve or thirteen, while at the same time they may become " difficult " with the mother. When such a state of affairs is evident, it may be welcomed, in spite

[1] *Brit. Journal Psychology*, Vol. XIII, 1922.

of the problems involved, for it suggests to the
psychologist that the girl's psycho-sexual development has at least progressed beyond the so-called
pre-genital stage—i.e. she is not wholly fixated in
the primitive relationship with the mother which
revolved round the experiences of feeding, cleanliness-training and toilet. That being so, the way
is more or less clear for her development to full
psycho-sexual maturity ; and in this last stage of
her psychological development, she may and should
make a claim for help on her father ; it is he who
can be of the greatest help to her now. In companionship with him (and with her brothers, if she
is fortunate enough to have brothers), she may be
imperceptibly prepared for the companionship of
marriage, for it is with a man that she will, it is
hoped, ultimately establish the major relationship
of her life. Close companionship with her mother
cannot offer this particular kind of preparation for
marriage. This, then, is the challenge to the
mother of an adolescent daughter : that she be
free from jealousy and possessiveness, in regard to
her daughter's relationship with her father ; and,
moreover, that she should let her go even further
afield in her search for guidance and help in her
emotional problems.

The mother of girls has certainly no easy task.
To stand aside with a quiet mind is often a much
more difficult undertaking than to take a part. In
the growing girl's difficulties, the mother will often
render the greatest service by being willing to let
her choose her own guide.

If the guide chosen is the father, then he too

has a difficult task to perform, for he has to see to it that this warmth of relationship and understanding which springs up between him and his daughter is transient in its intensity; that it does not become a " fixation "; that neither he nor his daughter become so emotionally involved in it, that she is hindered from establishing a satisfactory relationship with a man of her own generation, in whom, if marriage is to be successful, she must look to find, not a father, but a mate.

SEX INSTRUCTION AND GUIDANCE

So far, we have talked somewhat vaguely of " help " and " guidance ". What will this help and guidance consist in? Two main problems will be involved: first, what is the sex relationship? and second, the management of personal and of potentially sexual relationships. (The reader is reminded that we are at the moment dealing with the developing love-life of the adolescent girl, that is to say with only one, though perhaps the most important aspect of her life; it is not suggested that what follows covers all the " help and guidance " that she needs, as she grows from childhood to womanhood—far from it!)

Something has already been said about the giving of instruction in regard to menstruation. Many mothers feel that when they have given this instruction (in more or less vague terms) their duty as regards the teaching of the " facts of life " is fulfilled. It has scarcely begun to be performed. Girls and small children should know, as soon as they want to know, " where babies come from ":

the adolescent girl should know *how* babies come, and still more, what being married really means, physically and emotionally.

If, as many do feel, a mother feels she cannot possibly undertake such a task as this without embarrassment—either because her own attitude to sexual questions is uneasy, or because she is conscious of failures in her own marriage relationships which she feels she can neither ignore nor discuss—there is, nevertheless, still a great deal that she can do for her daughter. She can at least try to face the issues involved with genuine sincerity : to see things as they are ; and if she succeeds in this, she will at once be in a position to help, even if not directly. We are not discussing the psychology of mothers, and cannot therefore go at all deeply into the matter. But there is no doubt that although, as we have seen, much may happen in the psychological development of a girl from babyhood to make her relationship with her mother a difficult one, not all the difficulty comes from her side. As has been suggested, it is often the mother's own attitude to sexual life and experience which makes it impossible for her to discuss such matters in any helpful way with her daughter. Fear or shame in regard to her own sexual nature make her dread that her daughter should have any knowledge, let alone experience, in the matter. (Yet with strange inconsistency, she probably hopes that her girl will some day marry and have children ; but what depth of self-deception is sometimes concealed in that phrase " some day " !) A mother with this attitude is naturally incapable of helping her daughter. All she can do is to frighten or alienate her, according to the strength of the daughter's impulses and her confidence in them ; and this, tragically enough, in relation to matters—her love-life, her marriage and motherhood—which concern the most vital issues of happiness or wretchedness. In addition to this source of difficulty, there is another on the mother's side, which may be easier for her to tackle, and it is also related to the question of honesty, seeing things as they are. This is the difficulty that arises from the conscious or, more frequently unconscious, insincerity of mothers in their first attitude to their children. If babies were treated from the beginning as *persons*, and not, as so often, as cuddly *things*, the first step would be taken, from the mother's side at least, in the founding of a real and sincere relationship between herself and her children. And as time goes on, at every stage the mother's attitude should keep step with the child's development. Talk in the third person of the " mother wants Mary to be a good little girl " variety may be permissible before the child has grasped the significance of the personal pronouns, but how often do we find the same locutions being employed by mothers to big boys and girls whom no one else in their environment would dream of addressing in such a way. From such a small indication as this the child inevitably gets a feeling of unreality and sentimentality in her relationship with her mother ; and more than this, a feeling of not being properly respected as a person by mother, in the way other people, friends and teachers, respect her. Hence a reluctance to hear things from mother, which she could take readily from others. A block and an embarrassment of a really quite superficial character have entered into the relationship between mother and daughter which puts the mother out of reach as regards any power to give real help and guidance at a critical time. Thus the problem of sincerity or honesty, and the problem of respect for one's children as persons are seen to be closely connected; for honesty means a willingness to see things as they *are*, rather than as one would like them to be. Children *are* persons, not cuddly things, and the adolescent girl is in many ways a very complicated and elaborately, if not fully, developed person. It is not possible for a mother, or we might add, either parent, to make any real and helpful contact with a daughter of this age, except on the basis of complete sincerity. Only sincerity can give an adequate sense of security to the child in this parental relationship, which, as we have seen, contains within itself all the deeply repressed but still active conflicts of babyhood.

To return once more to this problem of putting young people in the way of the knowledge and guidance in regard to sex which they need at the age under discussion: as regards the facts, the matter is comparatively simple. The fuller and more complete these are, the greater will be the interest aroused. To describe the sex act, and leave out the story of all the physiological and endocrine activities involved in the mating of a man and his wife, and the producing and suckling of a child, is to reduce to a crude remark what might be an enthralling story. Books and diagrams can tell this story better than we can, perhaps, but at least we can let it be known (assuming all the subtle conditions of a satisfactory relationship as discussed above) that we appreciate the interest of the processes described and are willing to discuss them and answer any questions we can. There is no embarrassment when real interest has been aroused : and there is no doubt that the subject is supremely interesting.

My own experience in giving this information to adolescent girls—some of them very unstable—is that interest is invariable and the atmosphere of the interview is tense with it—even though rejection of the possibility of the experience of sexual life is absolute. " I think it's frightfully interesting, but simply awful," said one fifteen-year-old girl. No attempt to contest this judgment was made—only the comment : " Well, after all, you are not really ready for it as an experience yet, are you ? Perhaps in a few years' time it will seem more natural to you." Only a few months later she modified her judgment a little : " I do just begin to understand how it might be all right."

It is inevitable, and should be inevitable, that the girl takes this information personally, and relates it to her emotional life, as my fifteen-year-old did. To talk or act as if the intellectual interest of the subject were all we were concerned with is to be insincere again, and is probably evidence of that same fear and condemnation of sexuality, so common in the older generation, which has already been alluded to. It is essential that there be willing awareness of the connection between physical sexual feelings and the emotion of love, and that this connection be respected and not feared, if we are to be able in any way to give help to a girl who may be realizing this connection in her own experience for the first time. No probing, no questioning, is necessary. A sincere, unafraid, sensitive and respectful awareness will bring the questions from the other side; there is no need to ask them. In fact, to the anxious question: " What can I do to help my child in problems of love and potentially sexual friendships ? " the answer is usually : " Don't feel it incumbent on you to do anything; turn all your concern to the quiet realizing of what is happening in your child's mind and why it is happening." When this is the attitude in the mind of parent, head-mistress, or whoever it may be, the child for whom we are concerned will be enabled to *take* help and guidance, and this beyond anything that may be actually put into words.

THE SO-CALLED " SCHOOLGIRL CRUSH "

Before leaving this subject of the developing love-life of the adolescent girl, one must turn to another aspect of it, sufficiently common and, when it manifests itself, often so intense as to justify some real effort to understand it. This manifestation is accepted by some psychologists as " the homosexual phase of adolescence ", and by them it is regarded as essentially transient and more or less normal. They refer, of course, in the case of girls, to the " schoolgirl crushes " or " *grandes passions* "—" G.P.'s "—of girls for school-mistresses or older pupils ; and, in the case of boys, to the romantic attachments of older boys to younger ones.

In my opinion, this so-called homosexual phase is not an inevitable stage through which all boys and girls must pass, but is rather the product of our educational system, which as a general rule separates the sexes, and this frequently in boarding schools, at the very time when sexual love is dawning. What more natural, then, than that the boy should feel drawn to a younger boy who still bears some resemblance to a girl in the voice and delicacy of build belonging to his years, and the girl to an older girl, usually one characterized by athletic prowess, or (so very common) to the gym. mistress—often a woman of boyish type and build ? Curiously enough, while schoolgirl " crushes " are usually regarded by school authorities—sometimes with some unkindness—as silly rather than vicious, in boys' schools the romantic attachment, which usually has no conscious sexual factor in it at all, of an older boy to a younger one may be visited with almost savage severity. Yet, as we shall see, regarded from the psychological point of view, the girl's homosexual attachment may have far more ominous factors in it, from the point of view of her psycho-sexual development. In neither case are we dealing, usually, with any moral question at all, but simply with one of psycho-sexual development. But we have not yet begun to discuss the complexities of this question where girls are concerned.

As we have seen earlier in this discussion, it seems that the girl's psychological development from infancy to womanhood is a complicated and onerous affair, and in the course of its very earliest phases she is likely to be involved in intense conflicts between her dependence on her mother, her first love, and the rage and hate towards this same person, which are aroused by the inevitable demands and frustrations imposed by her on the baby, whose whole world of experience so far consists in feelings of pleasure or pain (un-pleasure). The child's craving for her mother's love and approval demands that she should find methods of dealing with these horrifying fantasies of rage and hate, and she does deal with them, with more or less success, by *repression* and by the expiatory methods of *projection*, whereby her own rage is conceived as being the mother's directed against herself, and *introjection*, which turns it directly on herself. All this, one must again remind one's readers, takes place inevitably, unconsciously, and at an age when there are no words in which emotional experience can find expression. But emotional experience it certainly is, confirmed again and again in the analysis of adults, and it is of a kind calculated to bring about what is known as *fixation* on the object of the experience, the mother. Where further experience has been favourable, particularly in the direction of the establishment of a happy relationship with the father, there may, however, be no unfortunate fixation on the mother. The girl will pass normally through the emotional upheavals of her adolescence —perhaps with a passing craze for the gym. mistress !—to the acceptance of a mate of the opposite sex with whom she can fulfil her emotional and sexual life as a wife and mother. In other cases, however, there is unmistakable evidence of mother-fixation, and one of the more obscure signs of this is the liability to form passionate attachments to school-mistresses and older girls and women. When such attachments do represent this state of affairs, they are serious, and need to be handled with extreme discretion, sympathy and tact. The connection between her love for her friend or mistress and her relationship with her mother is quite unrecognized by the girl. Often indeed she is passing through a " difficult " phase in regard to her mother, shown in her behaviour by irritability and criticism. She appears to resent the intimacy of her relationship with her mother, to be impatient of the latter's interest and concern in her affairs. This difficult relationship between the adolescent daughter and her mother is not characteristic of the mother-fixed girl alone; perhaps most girls pass through it to some extent. But in the mother-fixed girl there is likely to be a greater intensity of feeling, of hostility, resentment and withdrawal, combined with a profound need, mostly unconscious, for love, reassurance and approval. From this difficult ambivalent relationship such a girl will escape to an intense attachment to another woman, in which she can, as it were, start afresh, and find once more that association of perfect love : " mother " perfectly kind, and " baby " perfectly good, that existed before all the trouble of psychological growth began. It is, thus, in psychological language, a " transference " love, that is to say, it represents a transferring of feelings which originally belonged to the earliest personal relationships, analogous to that which occurs in the relationship between patient and doctor during a long course of psychological treatment. As such, it is fundamentally infantile in character, although fed with all the intensity of the adolescent girl's capacity for devotion and idealization ; for, in addition to these " transference " elements in the love, there is also at this age the awakening of that liability to " fall in love " which is a characteristic of all human beings throughout the greater part of their lives. Again, in psychological language, it is a regression : it is unconsciously an attempt to re-establish the golden age of babyhood. Many vivid illustrations of this were given in the film " Mädchen in Uniform " : for instance, the ecstasy of the motherless girl in receiving a present from the adored mistress, the intensity of ecstatic expectation in the dormitory as each girl waited for her good-night kiss. Hence we get a glimmer of why these schoolgirl passions so often carry a tragic element in them, and why they are transient and compulsively repeated. The golden age has passed and cannot be restored. The baby became too big for the womb, too big for the breast, and these transference loves carry always in them the infantile ambivalences, the unconscious battle between love and hate, which arose from these conflicts of desire with the demands of reality. It is because these " G.P.'s ", in their extreme development, represent such a regressive drive, that they strike one sometimes as almost psychotic (insane) in their intensity ; and they are thus no light matter to deal with. Ridicule is cruel and useless, in face of the compulsive longings and deep unconscious conflicts which such loves represent. The object of such adoration has a heavy responsibility. There is no cause for self-congratulation here ! But at the same time the adored one has an opportunity to help the adorer to renounce her unconscious infantile goals such as no one else has. Her task is as delicate as that of a psycho-analyst, but let her not attempt to be one ! Let her rather act on her realization of the significance of the situation, i.e. let her do all she can to change the relationship from a mother-child one to an equal one, and one based on reality, not on idealization. Shared interests, where these can be found, help in the first respect ; insisting on coming down off the pedestal, however and whenever opportunity offers, may help in the second : and in all contacts there should be a friendly and sympathetic demonstration of the realities of facts and experience. If the regressive drive we have described is very strong, this method of treatment may only succeed in shifting the burden of the responsibility to another woman or girl, to whom the passion of adoration will be transferred, because the needs it expresses have not been satisfied. If that is so, the first love may feel that she may nevertheless have done something to help her one-time adorer to give up the infantile mother-child relationship, even though for the moment she is seeking it elsewhere. She will at least have tried to demonstrate to her the possibility of an equal relationship, the only possible basis for a healthy and satisfying friendship.

It will perhaps be understood now why I spoke of the schoolgirl " Crush " being sometimes more ominous than the romantic friendships of boys. The latter are probably not often evidence of homosexual fixation. They are much more likely to be simply a question of *faute de mieux*. The schoolgirl crush, on the other hand, when it is of an intense and passionate kind, may lead to something like such fixation, especially if it is stimulated by its object. What we then get is an apparently homosexual fixation which is really a mother-fixation involving an arrest in psycho-sexual development. A girl who suffers an arrest of this kind may, however, do well in professional life. She may, indeed, find great happiness and satisfaction in certain professions, i.e. teaching, nursing and social work, her fixation working itself out in interest and concern for members of her own sex, in a manner quite compatible with mental health. Not all deviations from completely normal development (if there be such a thing) are disasters ! But she will find it very difficult to accept a relationship such as is involved in marriage, and she may unconsciously avoid opportunities that would open the prospect of marriage to her. While women preponderate so much numerically, this need not perhaps be regarded as a misfortune !

ADOLESCENCE AS " GROWING UP "

So far we have been considering the psychological aspects of adolescence as related to the developing love-life of girls. Let us in conclusion consider adolescence in its more general psychological aspect, simply as growing up : the transition from child-hood to womanhood. In what has been said, a good deal of attention has been paid to unconscious factors, having their origins in the earliest psycho-logical development of the child. In what follows we shall be dealing rather with conscious happen-ings, with the future rather than with the past.

Some girls are eager to grow up. Some are anxious to remain children. Some are torn between longing and fear in regard to being grown-up. Those in the first class are, as we have already suggested, likely to give considerable trouble to parents and people in authority during their adoles-cent years, and to become the healthiest women psychologically speaking. Those in the second class are likely to give least trouble in the early years of adolescence, but will be a constant source of anxiety when they reach the threshold of adult life. They are the girls who break down in their first posts, at twenty-one or so. At this stage they begin to have " nervous breakdowns ", seeking, consciously or unconsciously, by means of these, to retreat to the security of home again. Those in the third class make the most obvious demands for help ; their conflict is likely to become apparent during adolescence, manifesting itself in excessive emotional instability and inconsistent behaviour ; for instance, demanding privileges and shirking responsibilities, taking on enterprises and failing to carry them through. Let us consider these three types in rather more detail.

There is no doubt that the girl who is eager to claim grown-upness is often a trial to her elders.

Yet she should not be. There should be no
reluctance to let the young grow up. The days
when childhood was spoken of as the happiest
time of life are passing. Psychological investigation is showing us more and more that childhood
is anything but a time of ease and freedom. It is a
period of profound emotional experience, beginning
with the dawn of life, and there is little respite in it.
Children are at the mercy of so much and so many.
Even in the case of children surrounded by every
manifestation of care and affection, their wishes
and feelings are frequently and often inevitably
ignored and trampled on. Children have questions
asked them, and criticisms made of their behaviour,
which they will rightly regard as intolerable when
a few years older. Surely we should encourage the
young in their efforts to leave this stage of their
life behind them, and sympathize with their longing
to claim the privileges and immunities of adult life.
Their efforts in this direction may be very crude in
their manifestations. We may, for example, feel
outraged at the sight of lipstick and powder on a
fifteen-year-old face with which we have been
familiar from babyhood. But are we reasonable or
wise to protest ? Fundamentally it is an excellent
sign that the fifteen-year-old wants to be taken for
twenty-one, and mother's part in the affair, if she
is allowed one, should be that of sympathetic and
interested comrade in the æsthetics of make-up.
If she takes what is, I am afraid, the more usual
line, and either ridicules or scolds, nothing whatever
is gained after all ; for the inwardly sensitive, if
outwardly self-assured young thing is only outraged

by such treatment and her sense of alienation and hostility in regard to her mother is intensified, and this whether the make-up appears again or not. So from every point of view (including that of the artistic merit of the make-up!) an attitude of friendly interest is the profitable one. This is a small example of a kind which could be multiplied indefinitely. The principle is always the same. The adolescent girl, looking forward with courage and expectancy to adult life, should be encouraged all along the line, and respected in every experiment which she makes. Duties and obligations may indeed be indicated as inseparable from privileges, but indicated as part of the adventure, something more to risk, not as a deterrent. For example: "If you come in after eleven, will you do the locking-up and see that all's safe before you go up to bed?—then I can go to bed early with a quiet mind." Not: "Well, if you're not in till after eleven, you must jolly well see to the locking-up of everything yourself—you can't expect me to sit up for you." The first suggests a normal happening and full trust and sympathy; the second a fretful reproach and resentment. The first expresses a willingness to see a child grow up; the second fear and reluctance.

The child that does not want to grow up is a far greater problem; for something must already have gone wrong to bring this unnatural state of affairs about. There is also a possibility that we may be dealing here with constitutionally poor material from the point of view of personality and character. If analysis of such a child were possible, it would probably be found that at every step demanding advance, there were difficulties—in the establishment of breast feeding, in weaning, with the birth of another child, first attendance at school, etc. These difficulties are forgotten as the child develops, perhaps into a docile, well-behaved girl, and she may even come to be regarded as the model of all a schoolgirl should be, loyal and keen in all school activities, without a thought beyond. School and home are her secure little world, held fast in fear of the future and its demands for new adjustments. I am not of course suggesting that all model schoolgirls are Peter Pans; rather that some Peter Pans are model schoolgirls, and the disappointment is all the greater when they break down on the threshold of adult life, as such Peter Pans tend to do, when they first meet real demands for responsibility, courage and forgetfulness of self.

In other cases the fear of growing up may be so intense as to cause obvious difficulties throughout childhood and girlhood, every change being resisted with anxiety, as in the case of a child who wept over giving up socks, and the lengthening of her frocks, clinging to old familiar clothes, and rejecting new ones. Such cases, however, are so clamant for help that they are more likely to get it in one way or another. It is the cases of what one may call occult Peter Panism, such as I have described, that miss detection until too late to avoid breakdown under the strain of grown-up life. Similarly, those children who are torn between desire and fear in regard to getting older are likely to throw up signs of their disquietude in behaviour difficulties of a more complicated kind than a mere claiming of age by smoking, making-up or the like. When there is conflict between opposing wishes, conscious or unconscious, symptoms are apt to develop, and these may be infinitely varied. Some of the emotional instability which is regarded as characteristic of adolescence may, in fact, have its source in this conflict, rather than in any gland imbalance, and this fact should always be borne in mind.

To return to a suggestion made earlier in this discussion : Whether or not there is, as Dr. Ernest Jones suggests, an actual recapitulation during adolescence of the emotional conflicts and adjustments of those notorious " first five years ", there is no doubt that a girl does during adolescence carry through a complicated process of adjustment and readjustment, both physical and emotional, at the end of which, if she is successful, she is ready to assume the responsibilities and the independence of adult life.

If Dr. Jones's suggestion is borne in mind, it should, moreover, help us to comprehend and forbear with some of the vagaries of adolescence, which might otherwise provoke irritation and ridicule. The latter is often thought of as " bracing ", but actually it is likely to be deeply upsetting to a child who is coping with emotional difficulties which she is far from understanding. The access of puritanism, for instance, which some girls assume—perhaps for a very short period—may be recognized as the (unconscious) effort of her super-ego (or ego-ideal) to contend, by over-reaction, with the strong instinctual impulses which must accompany sexual development. This puritan or idealistic or religious phase may in due course yield to another phase, apparently very inconsistent, of lethargy or feverish pleasure-seeking. To the psychologist there is no necessary assumption of instability or deterioration here. All it may mean is the passing of some deep unconscious stress, and a temporary, inevitable reaction. It is important to remember that most of these adjustments and readjustments during this stormy period are made of necessity and unawares. If we, the " older and wiser ", can, through comprehension, recognize the inner necessity to the girl of some of these apparently exaggerated and perhaps irritating phases, we shall find it possible to refrain from criticism, which can, in the circumstances, only alienate and exasperate ; and by our very forbearance it may be that we shall be able to provide much-needed reassurance.

THE EDUCATION OF THE ADOLESCENT GIRL

It is not within my province to enter upon a discussion of the scholastic education of the adolescent girl ; but in view of her special difficulties one would like to make a plea for some implicit recognition of these in educational schemes. The education of girls is, compared with that of boys, a comparatively recent development ; and it has, very naturally, been evolved in imitation of the traditions of male education. While a total cleavage between the ideals and methods of boys' and girls' education would be a disaster, and quite as unnatural as the present imposition of masculine educational traditions on girls, yet it should surely be possible to modify the education of girls during adolescence in such a way as, on the one hand, to relieve unnecessary and useless strain (e.g. compulsory games, examinations where not required for professional purposes, long hours of home-work), and, on the other, to provide some more explicit preparation for life *as a woman*, that is, as a wife and mother. Neither of these factors seem, as far as one can judge, to be taken much into account in the education provided by secondary schools. Yet both are of paramount importance to the health and happiness of the schoolgirl, and of the woman of the future.

CONCLUSION

Perhaps it will be thought that in what I have written I have laid too much stress upon the difficulties of adolescence, and that I demand more sympathy for the adolescent girl than she needs, or than is good for her. I do not think so. Medical and psychological training, as a result of which I come to be contributing this chapter, have in the course of years but confirmed that conviction of the intensity of the emotional upheaval of adolescence, which makes me remember now how once I stood in my bedroom cubicle at school, and cried to myself: " *Never* will I forget what it is like to be fifteen! "

IV. PERSONALITY DEVIATIONS IN CHILDREN

By CLIFFORD ALLEN, M.D., M.R.C.P., D.P.M.,
INSTITUTE OF MEDICAL PSYCHOLOGY

IV. PERSONALITY DEVIATIONS IN CHILDREN

BY CLIFFORD ALLEN, M.D., M.R.C.P., D.P.M.,
INSTITUTE OF MEDICAL PSYCHOLOGY

THE popular idea of a personality tends to approximate somewhat with those views regarding it which were formulated by our Victorian ancestors. They thought that a personality was inherited as such and was not easily altered. Much as one boy inherited red hair and a stately mansion or another inherited black hair and nothing but poverty, so it was believed that a merciful Providence endowed each child with an appropriate personality. If he inherited a " good " personality the consequence was that he worked hard and in due time prospered and married his employer's daughter. If he was unfortunate enough to inherit a " bad " personality then the resulting weakness showed itself in squandering his substance in riotous living and reaching the workhouse by way of Carey Street. In spite of this rigid idea that the personality was inherited more or less complete, many who held this view had some faint idea that it could be modified by appropriate measures. These measures were to be taken by the parents and later by the schoolmaster. Their kindly (or, more usual, unkindly) ministrations were capable of modifying the personality to some slight degree and usually took the form of not sparing the rod. Apart from this slight capacity for modification the personality was regarded as unmalleable and not easily moulded.

It is not strange that such a rigid and unnatural view of the personality should have been abandoned and a more biological one formulated to replace it. What, one might ask, is the modern view of the nature of the personality? The answer is that the personality is regarded as an organ, or perhaps a collection of organs much as the physical body is a collection of organs, and that far from being inherited as a complete and developed structure it grows and suffers all the modifications which environment, disease, and so on, can inflict.

Now an organ (or a collection of organs) is developed merely for one purpose—that is in order that the organism may adjust itself to the world in which it must live. The eyes were not developed for the pleasure of looking at things but in order that the animal should be aware of danger at a distance and make suitable adjustments before the charging buffalo (or whatever danger it may be) should be able to inflict damage upon the spectator. Just in the same way the more complicated organ, the personality, has developed in order that the child may be able to adjust itself to the world around it. It is a collection of responses to the situations which occur and far from being any mystical inheritance it must naturally grow by slowly adding one response to another until the collection becomes large enough to give a correct response to any situation which may reasonably be regarded as likely to occur.

We now arrive at the difference between that which constitutes a good personality and a bad one. A good personality is formed by the development of suitable reactions which are entirely appropriate to the situation. The possessor of a good personality is never at a loss and is always able to cope with any situation, no matter how bizarre it may be. He is able to make the correct emotional adjustments in every case. The possessor of a " bad " personality is in quite a different position. His reactions and responses are not suitable and he tends to have but one type of response, to which he clings like a leech and uses to meet every situation. These responses would be quite valuable if they were used in the appropriate situation, but if they are used on any and every occasion, sooner or later they bring their possessor to disaster. Thus we find that children tend to fall into groups, such as the shy child, the over-aggressive child and so on. Now shyness, or a withdrawing reaction, is a valuable mode of response to certain situations. Obviously those who are shy, or reluctant to make contact, will avoid the dangers which will fall to the lot of those fools who rush in too gladly. Similarly a reaction such as over-aggressiveness is a very valuable one if it is used in the right situation. The over-aggressive reaction will frighten off enemies before they dare attack and so avoid many encounters which might prove disastrous.

Nevertheless, if but *one* reaction is used all the time then many situations which should prove beneficial to the child will be passed by without profit. The shy child will regard even those who are kindly disposed to him as enemies, and thus he will fail to make any happy social contacts—whereas the over-aggressive child will reach the same miserable state by frightening off those who would have been his friends had he not been so terrifying.

The utilization of one single reaction is bad enough as a personality fault, but there is still a worse one. This is giving the *wrong* response in all situations. Children of this type are not responding to the current environment at all but to some other surroundings in which they have found themselves in the past. The result of such a grave personality deviation as this is to produce an odd, queer child who fails to fit in anywhere.

These descriptions are of the more or less developed personality, but one might with reason say: "You have said that one is not born with a completely developed personality. How is this psychic organ developed and how can one prevent it from becoming diseased and unhealthy?" The development of the personality and the gradual growth to the complete structure is by no means simple. It might be supposed that the personality would grow solely as the result of experience modifying those instinctive modes of reaction which *are* inherited, such as fear of loud noises and so on. This must be the way in which animals develop such personalities as they may have. It is, however, a very slow way of forming a collection of responses and it is far from being entirely safe. If we have to experience every situation to which we must learn to respond obviously we shall have to face difficult and dangerous ones to know what we should do in every case. Doubtless the child would be destroyed long before it developed any personality at all. Nevertheless a child does develop some of its personality in this way, and the endless curiosity and capacity for exploration, which every child shows, helps it in this direction. It burns itself and consequently knows in future that fire is painful and best avoided, teases the dog and learns that dogs bite and so on. This path to the perfect personality is a slow, painful and dangerous one and it is fortunate that the child has quicker means of development than by exclusively personal experience in every case. This means of development is to be found in the fact that the child has at hand its parents, who have already developed (or should have developed) appropriate personalities and so constitute a fund of experience from which the child can draw ready-made reactions without any danger at all. There has always been a vague idea that the child models itself upon its parents, but exactly how it does it has only recently been known. We now believe that at the time when the child wants to put everything into its mouth so, at the same time, does it repeat its behaviour psychically.

It moulds itself upon its parents by a curious reaction to them which is known as introjection. By this means it absorbs them physically and identifies itself so completely with them that it treats itself as though it, itself, were the parent. The love and hate which it has felt for the parent in the past have now been reversed on to the child because by completely identifying itself with its parents it is unable to direct it elsewhere. This is not mimicry, which is merely conscious imitation and can be ceased at will. Introjection is much more subtle and very difficult to observe; it is entirely unconscious and is not under the power of the child's volition at all. Probably when this identification with the parents occurs it is not easily modified.

It is obvious then that if the child is going to absorb all of its mother's, and, later, all of its father's responses, *in toto*, with one fell swoop, it will be saved a great deal of trouble and danger in so doing. No doubt this is the biological reason for this strange process of introjection. One might conclude that the formation of the personality was a simple matter since, if the parent had made some response to a situation, the child, by identifying itself with the parent, might now be expected to give the same response. No doubt this does happen in a large number of cases, and one frequently finds that a child is afraid of, let us say, cows merely because its mother is afraid of them and has shown fear in the child's presence. This may occur in spite of the fact that cows have never menaced it in any way and it has never seen them do anything fearful. The child has just acquired the response, without reasoning, from its mother.

This would be a convenient manner in which to construct a personality, were it not that the process of introjection is complicated by the fact that the child loves and hates the parent with whom it identifies itself. This may be considered unfortunate, but it is probable that introjection would not occur at all but for the intense emotion which the child feels for its parent. Once it has made the psychic absorption and identified itself with its mother it *must* turn the emotion which it felt for her upon itself; moreover, it has now in its mind a kind of "psychic mother" which is always in its mind and from which it can never escape. The greater the emotion it had for its mother the worse it will suffer. If it hated its mother savagely then this introjected mother will treat it as cruelly as it would have treated her. Moreover, it has to accord with such as were her standards. Perhaps formerly it was fond of playing with dirt and enjoyed forbidden pleasures, but now it has this "mental mother" in its mind which says with the harsh voice of the real mother, "No, dirty," and it dare not break the law.

One might think that by this time the child has had ample opportunity to form its personality, in spite of the fact that all this has occurred at an early age, but it is not so. The personality is still developing even after introjection and the child is constantly making responses with that amount of personality which it has developed while adding to its personality at the same time. The process then is far from simple. Moreover, the child has up to this time been responding purely in response to the pleasure which it obtained from suitable reactions, now, however, it begins to respond to the reality of its environment. It has to learn to curb its wishes for immediate pleasure to gain some greater but future delights. Everyone has observed even the most spendthrift child saving its Saturday pennies, in spite of all temptations, in order to buy the toy engine which it covets, and it would be absurd to pretend that the reactions which will eventually form its personality are not added to and developed in this way.

When, during the earlier part of its childhood, the small child tends to direct its energies to obtaining pleasure it is essential that it should be allowed to do so to a reasonable degree, since to thwart its desires too ruthlessly may have a profound effect on its future personality. It is believed that some children who are weaned too early, too late, or too abruptly, miss the pleasurable sensations which they should have had in suckling at the breast and consequently grow into disagreeable and envious folk, always seeking what they have not got and eager to wrench from their neighbours the possessions which they feel they have missed. Again, if during the infancy the child is fussed too much about the routine of its bowels, if its mother over-emphasizes the importance of this function, there is danger of the child developing into the over-moral adult who makes his own and others' lives a constant misery by his scruples and worries about things which really do not matter in the least.

One can influence the child in the direction of developing satisfactory responses (or a " good " personality) both in this earlier stage of pleasure-seeking and in the later stage of response to reality by making the environment such that its natural desires will lead it into the right response. In the pleasure-seeking stage the child is able to overcome its desires in three ways. It can force these wishes out of its mind and by repressing them forget that it ever had them. This will not necessarily influence its personality, although it may do so if the forces which are pushing the wish out of its thoughts become weakened. Another way by which it can deal with the wish is to symbolize it, and this is much more satisfactory since it allows some satisfaction as well as being more social than other ways. An instance of this is when a child who wishes to play with dirt symbolizes it by painting and paints the garden fence. This is a good reaction and allows the wish to be gratified without being antisocial. The third way it can respond to a wish which is forbidden is by doing exactly the opposite. An example of this is seen when such a child instead of playing with dirt becomes excessively clean. Although this is a social response it carries with it a certain danger, since the child may spend so much time on cleanliness that life becomes a burden and the incessant washing an illness.

In order to develop a satisfactory personality therefore the child must have a number of conditions. Firstly it must have parents who have good personalities and satisfactory responses themselves, so that when it moulds itself on them (or introjects them) it will have a store of reliable responses obtained from them. If the parents suffer from some defect themselves then there is a likelihood that the child will acquire the same defect by the very fact that it has moulded itself upon the parent. A shy parent tends to have a shy child and so on. It is very important that the parent should be free from nervous or mental diseases, since there is a possibility that the child may acquire the reactions which characterize the disease and so lay the foundations for the future development of the illness. We know that a husband and wife living in close intimacy may influence each other and that the wife may acquire the husband's delusions— how much more is it possible that the malleable mind of the child may be infected by the delusions of an insane parent or the nervous aches and pains of a neurotic one? The next essential for the development of a good personality is that the child should be allowed every faculty to make contact with reality and acquire unaided all those reactions it may and build upon those which it has acquired from its parents. Now this is often prevented by over-anxious parents who are afraid that the child will come to some disaster. It is not unusual to find that parents who have lost their first child over-protect the next one so that this child is never allowed out alone, never plays with other children, and when later on it is called upon to face the world it has to learn those reactions which it would have acquired with ease had it been allowed to do so. This is a biological fact and is proved by the case of kittens. They instinctively chase moving objects and if they encounter mice at an early age know how to kill them. If they never see any mice until they are older they lose the instinctive knowledge and have to *learn* how to kill them. In the same way children who have not been allowed to indulge in little fights and to stand up for themselves will later have to learn laboriously how to do so.

The third essential in the development of a good personality is that the child should have every encouragement, in its environment, to develop pleasure in social responses. Obviously, if it obtains pleasure from antisocial responses then it will grow up antisocial. One of the worst thieves which the writer has ever had to treat was a young man whose first theft was to take the milk-bottle off the doorstep of a neighbour The family applauded instead of telling the child to take it back. He went on doing little thefts and was always being praised for his cleverness in doing so. The thefts grew and grew into more serious ones until the family suddenly became alarmed. By this time the matter was grave and the boy was a confirmed thief.

The danger of allowing the personality to deviate, to allow one reaction to become the permanent response, is that sooner or later it leads either to major or minor disasters. Those who suffer from the less marked deviations tend to become unhappy misfits, the unfortunate malcontent who drift through life missing the happiness they should have had and spreading an aura of misery around them. Those who have more serious deviations and make entirely wrong reactions have even more disastrous terminations. It is these unfortunates who become the neurotics, the insane, tramps and prostitutes. Doubtless it would be easy to dismiss this as the scaremongering fears of the academic psychologist if proof to the contrary were not so easily forthcoming. The investigations of Kasanin and Veo show this clearly. These investigators took a group of young people who had become insane, traced the schools which they had attended, and enquired of their teachers concerning the personalities of the young men and girls as observed by them when they were under their care. It was found that 50 per cent. of the children were abnormal when at school. Actually 25 per cent. were described as being " odd and queer " (meaning that they made inappropriate reactions). The other 25 per cent. were of the shy, withdrawing " nobody " type. Now it is quite probable that the other 50 per cent. who seemed normal to the teachers might have also shown some abnormality had they been examined by a trained psychologist instead of laymen, however interested and observant they were, and it is not unreasonable to presume that, had the children who were noticed to be developing bad, unsuitable or wrong reactions been treated and these reactions corrected, they might never have become insane.

The commonest personality defect is shown by the shy child. This child has developed such a personality either by being the unfortunate possessor of parents who were themselves shy and so has modelled himself upon an imperfect model, or else has never been allowed to make real contact with other children and so has no proper experience with reality. The timidity which is often found accompanying shyness and which is frequently indistinguishable from it is usually due to the fact that it has had a great deal of hostility aroused, usually by unsuitable treatment, and has overcome this hatred to such an extent that far from being aggressive it is shy and timid.

This child shows its characteristic reaction at an early age. It usually prefers to play alone and never plays much with other children even in inviting circumstances. At parties it at once appears to be " out of it " and shrinks awkwardly into corners while the other children are romping in the centre of the room. It may even look at the games with longing eyes, but it is much too shy and timid to take a part in them. This is the child that is often brought to the psychologist, or at least makes itself conspicuous, because of its fears. It is afraid of big dogs, although it has never received any harm from one, and the whistle of a railway engine reduces it to a shuddering jelly. Its fears often occur again in its sleep and its nightmares arouse it when its more stolid brothers are fast asleep. The dark is more fearful to this child than it is to others and a journey into a dark room to fetch something is more terrifying than it is possible to imagine. When it goes to school it shows its withdrawing reaction again. It does not join in the football or cricket, but wanders off into quiet corners of the playing fields where it will not be worried by the presence of others. In class it fails to gain the distinctions which it should because it is too shy and too timid to show its knowledge. If the master (who appears to it like an enormous giant eager to threaten it with terrifying punishments) is able to gain its confidence, and allay its fears to some extent, a child of this type may show more intelligence than rougher and less timid children. Usually children who show this shy, withdrawing reaction learn to read easily, and having discovered literature they use it as the perfect escape from the harsh world. They are often omnivorous in their tastes and will read so extensively that if their parents knew the field of their studies they would be surprised. It is more often fiction than text-books that they read, but sometimes children of this type do take a surprising interest in their work and then they do brilliantly —except that their lives become miseries because other children look on them as abnormalities and " swats " and ill-treat them. This withdrawing reaction which is characterized by shyness is particularly devastating inasmuch as it makes it impossible for the child to improve it itself. The reaction tends to form a vicious circle and get worse and worse. This is particularly so when the child discovers, for example, sex. Children who show this reaction never discuss sex with other children and never hear anything about it. The consequence is that they never acquire the rudimentary ideas which most children have (until they become old enough to acquire sexual knowledge through books). When they discover, as most children do, sex through masturbation, they form all sorts of abnormal ideas about what they are doing, and having a vague idea that it is wrong they acquire an abnormal sense of guilt. This in itself tends to make the child more seclusive and shy, so that it has less chance of learning that what it is doing is normal and of losing the guilty feelings. Again, shy children have less chance of contact with other children of the opposite sex. They tend to be thrown back on to their mothers or fathers for someone to love. The result of this is only too often that they become abnormally attached to the parent and even develop homosexuality as the result. Here, again, the feeling of guilt is aroused and the child prevented still further from developing normal sexuality. With their shyness there is often a genuine sense of deprivation that they cannot mix more freely, and often such children make real efforts to do so. They are usually gauche in their efforts and their shyness makes them nervous. It is this child who attempts to be social in such an awkward way that it is likely to raise laughter, with, of course, disastrous results to its efforts and feelings.

One might ask what the results in after life are with such children. They are as disastrous as those in childhood. It finds puberty a strain because of the strong emotions which it cannot express and the fact that the process appears mysterious because it is too shy to ask what is happening. After this the young man emerges who is still just as timid and shy. If he falls in love he is far too shy ever to approach the object of his desires and, although his feelings may be boiling over, he will only worship her from afar. If he is supremely daring he will make some approach which is likely to meet with little success because of its very clumsiness. Having been hurt by a girl, the young man abandons women and tends to develop into a lonely individual who lives a miserable life brooding on what he might have done or what he might have had if fate had been kinder. Sometimes he sublimates his emotions in art, but even then he tends to be the shy solitary painter or writer who lives alone in dreary solitude. If he does not become an artist, then too often he becomes a solitary wanderer, if he has money perhaps an explorer, but if he has none he may sink to the level of a tramp trudging from one workhouse to another. Although this is, perhaps, a dreary picture it is the rosier side of the termination of the extreme withdrawal which the shy child shows. The darker side is the case where the child grows into the extreme recluse who broods upon his fate continually and whose solitariness leads inevitably to some form of abnormal sexuality. He feels that the world is hostile to him, develops ideas of persecution which grow into delusions, and result in definite insanity. Often this does not show itself for years—mainly because such people do not form any contacts where it might be discovered—but eventually it shows itself in a bizarre act which leads to some custodial treatment. As Kasanin and Veo showed, this is but the illness whose long shadow could have been noticed in childhood had anyone looked for its presence.

The exact opposite to the shy withdrawing reaction is an aggressive one. This is a healthy reaction, but if there is an excess of aggression which passes out of the patient's control there is a danger of the reaction becoming unhealthy. The aggressive reaction brings the child into contact with other children, and the aggression which it arouses in them forms a corrective if the child is able to play with them at an early age.

An over-aggressive reaction may be caused by

the fact that the child has modelled itself upon parents who are themselves aggressive; but they may have allowed it to develop over-aggressive reactions by their very passivity (if they are easy-going people), and the fact that the child has found that aggression is an easy way of obtaining what he wants has made it choose this reaction to the exclusion of others.

The child which is going to use the aggressive reaction for the rest of its life shows its choice at an early age. This is the reaction which makes the child lie on the pavement and scream because its mother will not buy it the expensive toy engine which it has seen in a shop window. It is this child who bawls until the home resounds because it discovers that the sweet is not what it expected for lunch. It will rush at its parent and bite because it cannot obtain its own way. (Of course every child will make some show of temper at some time or other, but it must be remembered that it is the *persistent* use of *one type of reaction* which we have defined as a personality deviation and it is not a solitary act which is dangerous but a constant repetition of the same sort of reaction.) The over-aggressive child terrorizes its brothers and sisters —if they are not too big to allow it—and is always willing to start a fight over something trivial—like the possession of a sand-castle and so on.

When children who show this reaction go to school they usually succeed in making their presence felt by their savage assaults. Their over-aggressiveness tends to lead them into bullying and consequently unpopularity. With this over-aggressiveness, and usually the cause of it, goes hostility to the parents. This the child turns on to the masters and he is the boy who leads the riots against the weak form-master and even raises his fists to the stern one. As he grows older he becomes more and more hostile to authority. Because his style of reaction forces him into contact with others he tends to learn of sex at an early age. He looks on sex as a form of rebellion against his elders and indulges in it with all the joy of revolt. He it is that teaches the other boys about masturbation, whether they want to know about it or not. His over-aggressiveness often results in his expulsion from school, and if he goes to a university, in wild adventures which terminate his academic career by being " sent down ".

This over-aggressiveness often prevents him settling down into a satisfactory worker in whatever post he occupies later. He is the type of man who is ag'in the Government, whatever it may be. He quarrels with those in authority and bullies those who are under him. His hostility and bullying make him unpopular and, feeling it, he becomes surlier and more aggressive. Such a personality deviation does not often lead to mental illness, but it may do so. A case of this type of reaction was once under the writer's care. He was a young man who had shown this over-aggressiveness at school, with the result that he was extremely unpopular. When he left school he became a cadet in the Navy. As soon as he joined he obtained a copy of the King's Regulations and studied this and Naval Law. He did this not from any laudable interest in his career, but merely in order that he should have the power to trip up his superiors when they gave him an order or acted in any way he disliked. Needless to say, he was extremely unpopular in every ship in which he served and at last decided that the Navy was an unsuitable career. He obtained work in another capacity, but was still very aggressive. On one occasion he reacted excessively to a man, who trod accidentally upon his foot, while he was listening to a concert in a London concert hall, and the result was almost a fight in the midst of a symphony! This young man became worse and worse until he developed a definite mental illness which necessitated treatment.

Another personality defect which causes its owner endless trouble is what might be called an obstinate mulish reaction. This, like the other, may be caused by the child introjecting, or modelling itself upon, its parents who, themselves, show unreasoning obstinacy. It is more usual that obstinacy is the outward sign of hostility to the parents or, of course, a reaction which the child has found will conquer opposition and which it has developed to excess.

Like the other reactions, the child tends to develop it early. Children of this type are those who hold their breath in screaming fits and who obstinately refuse to learn the functions of the toilet at the behest of their mothers. They can be led but not driven, and any attempt to drive them arouses such a display of mulishness that their parents are driven to despair. When they go to school they will often display a truly astonishing refusal to learn things which they do not like. This often leads to the teacher becoming annoyed with their apparent stupidity and to showing anger with them. This, of course, increases the tension, so that the child becomes even more obstinate. This child will sometimes mix well with other children, and as long as no attempt is made by the others to coerce it, it will play happily enough. The obstinate reaction makes it difficult for it to become either a leader or a follower, so that it rarely distinguishes itself in the community. If its reaction is turned to advantage (as it may be by a wise teacher) such a child will achieve results which could only be achieved by unremitting work and will leave the more brilliant intellectual child, who has less determination, far behind.

This is the reaction which makes the child set its mind on one particular career, and when it leaves school it will turn all its energies to achieving this aim. This is, of course, satisfactory providing that it is the sort of career to which it is suited and which is within its intellectual capacities, but will lead to disaster if it is not. Developed to excess, this obstinate reaction gives the possessor less chance of success than a more flexible reaction. It allows no adjustment to changing circumstances. In itself therefore it may lead to emotional and financial disaster which lands the possessor into misery and sometimes insanity.

Another type of reaction which is very frequently overlooked in children is that of over-conscientiousness. The child who presents this response gives the appearance of being a " model child ", but it is really presenting signs of illness. Children should not be models, but children. This type of reaction is produced in a family where there is an air of fussiness and over-scrupulousness. The parents tend to be either " born fussers " and worry about the slightest thing, so that the child lives in an atmosphere of parental criticism, or else the parents are those excessively religious sort of people who magnify everything into a sin and the child lives in constant fear of breaking human and divine laws almost by the act of breathing. The constant correction invariably brings about a feeling of hostility to the parents, and when it introjects them or models itself upon them this hostility turns on to the child itself, with the result that it becomes timid, frightened, and excessively scrupulous. Although this reaction appears like all the others at an early age, it is not easy to observe it as early as the others. Nevertheless, the guilt which is constantly in the child's mind and the fears which its tiny transgressions arouse soon make it a worried child and disturb its sleep with terrible dreams of appalling retribution which it feels it must have incurred by its incredible iniquity. Besides night-terrors the child who shows this type of reaction is worried in the daytime, and it is particularly fearful of new environments lest it break some unknown code of morals. It is this type of child who worries excessively about things which other children do with a light heart—the stealing of sugar or the neighbour's fruit appears to it to be next to murder in sinfulness. It is this child who is always held up, when it is small, as an example. It never falls into duck-ponds and comes home covered with mud, but sits at home with its hands nicely washed and its hair neatly brushed, quietly developing what will later appear as a neurosis.

This child finds school a tremendous ordeal. Its over-scrupulousness leads it to work harder—much harder—than other children, so that it pleases its teachers, and of course it never misbehaves under any circumstances. It tends to develop into the teacher's favourite and when the end of the term comes it is moved into the next form. Here it finds that it has to compete with older and cleverer children, but its over-scrupulousness drives it on to do so. By superhuman efforts it at last reaches the top of the class and passes ahead of its older competitors. Now one might think that it could rest on its laurels, but its over-scrupulousness is its downfall. It is promoted into the next class. Here it meets still older and still cleverer children, but its psychological condition will not allow it to realize that its task is an impossible one. It is driven on to overcome these still more appalling conditions, and it strives on until it either collapses with a neurosis or the teacher sees that it is breaking down, and relaxes the strain by stopping its promotion. It is not only in the fact that it tends to rise to forms beyond its capacity which tests this child's personality. Its intense work is often resented by the other children, who show hostility to it and reward its intellectual superiority by demonstrating their physical strength. It becomes miserably bullied. It dare not cease to work because its over-conscientiousness would make its life a misery, and yet to work like it does leads to endless attacks from other children.

When this child discovers sex he is again faced with the same problem created by his over-scrupulousness. Other children indulge in sex and take it as a part of life. They never worry much about masturbation, whether it is indulged in as a solitary experience or with others. When the over-scrupulous child discovers it, however, he is faced with terrible conflicts. He feels constantly driven on by the sexual urge, which is made stronger by the fact that he tries to overcome it, but his over-scrupulousness and his conscientious attitude make him feel that this is a terrible sin which he must abolish at all costs. His life becomes a constant fight to subdue the sexual instinct.

If this child has intellectual powers, then it is likely that he will succeed in making his way—unless he is too ill and breaks down before he does so. He will make everybody's life a misery, however, by his fussiness and usually arouses contempt by it. If he has not got a fine intellect he will almost invariably collapse under the strain which his reaction arouses.

It might be thought that all this is but the gloomy picture which a psychologist paints to frighten parents. It is not so and the cases which show evidence of the obsessional neurosis—that is, people who are obsessed with ideas of dirt, who have to go back five times to see that the gas is turned off, who worry lest they forget to shut the front door, etc.—all have a history of this type. The writer knows of a family in which the father is afflicted with obsessional ideas regarding religion, so that the trivialities of religious observance have become his whole life.

The mother is an hysteric and has ruled the family with a rod of iron by means of her neurosis. The eldest son is an obsessional neurotic and spends his life worrying about whether he has turned off taps and so on. The middle son is normal, except for an excess of anxiety, and has achieved success. The youngest son is another obsessional neurotic and has had a miserable life because of his illness. There is no doubt in such a case that the children were brought up in a wrong atmosphere and that they introjected their father with all his illness *en bloc*.

One of the saddest types of child is that which is the " odd queer child ". Now it has been pointed out that a personality deviation is mainly characterized by the fact that the child is constantly responding with one reaction which it uses to the exclusion of others. Often this reaction may be used in the right situation and so is the correct one, although, of course, often it is incorrect. With the odd queer child we find that it is always responding by the *wrong reaction*. It is this which gives its oddness and its apparent queerness. It is odd and queer because it is never responding correctly. Now the constant repetition of one type of reaction tends towards the neurosis—hysteria or obsession or what not. But the production of the wrong type of reaction on every occasion tends to approximate with insanity. Insanity is itself but a wrong reaction. It is not surprising therefore that Kasanin and Veo found that 25 per cent. of those children who become insane in later life are comprised of these odd queer children who are sometimes said by their teachers to behave as though they were mad.

Children who show this type of inappropriate reaction are produced either by the fact that one or both of their parents are insane and the child has introjected their personalities (with the insane reactions) *in toto*, or, more commonly, that they have been forced to face an environment which is hostile to them, and to which they have not been able to make proper adjustments. The unwanted child, the child whose parents wanted one of another sex, and so on, tend to compose this group.

Children who show this type of reaction often display it early but it is not understood. A mother of such a child told the writer that she noticed that when it was a baby whilst being bathed it held itself stiffly and resisted her. Instead of treating this child with especial love and care, this behaviour aroused her hostility.

Since they have difficulty in finding the right reaction children of this type are nearly always solitary children and do not play with other children, but if they do, the other children do not understand them and so " rag " and bully them. The child's behaviour is often difficult to understand even at an early age. It is this child who gives away all the family crockery to the dustman, empties the kettle on the fire, or (like a case of the writer's) puts all the watches and clocks in the house down the lavatory ! When he goes to school the boy who shows this type of reaction usually has a rough time. He appears clumsy and awkward and, of course, he is a failure at games. In his work he is more likely to show flashes of brilliance (when he more or less accidentally does react correctly) than any steady rhythm.

135

He is always a lonely figure and regarded both by masters and boys as being eccentric (or even mad). While other young Apollos score centuries before admiring relatives, the child of this type will be found alone and friendless at the edge of the throng. This child has an astonishing capacity of wearing his clothes so that they look ridiculous ; no matter how expensive they may be, they always appear as though they were not made for him and are dreadfully untidy. He buttons up his waistcoat unevenly and ties his tie inside out at the age when other boys are beginning to exhibit fancy silk socks and commence creasing their trousers. The writer has under his care at the present time a young man who shows all these characteristics. He always comes for treatment carrying a little walking-stick with a dog's-head handle, his clothes never seem to fit him, and are always put on wrongly in some way. When this child discovers sex he again behaves in an unusual way. Either he develops excessive guilt about it, or else he behaves in a way which gives the impression that he is quite callous to the whole matter. This is never really the case with such children and they are most exquisitely sensitive and capable of extreme suffering. Usually their adolescent love-affairs are more disastrous than most because of their peculiar appearance and behaviour, which scares off the girl for whom they feel so strongly.

When this child grows into early manhood he usually experiences great difficulty in finding a niche in the social system into which he can fit happily. He is often forced into positions which are really quite unworthy of his intellectual abilities because he is never able to develop the *savoir faire* (that is, the correct reactions) which would enable him to obtain a better post. If he goes to a university he is usually distinguished by being an odd, peculiar, eccentric person who has few friends and spends his time studying something which other people think is of no earthly use. Later he develops into a gross eccentric and this may develop into real insanity. It is this type which furnishes the prophets and quacks, the founders of new faiths and arts, the devotees of pseudo-sciences. Too often, however, the world of illusion becomes too strong and they forsake the world of reality, which they have found so unhappy, for it. They develop the delusions that they are Christ or feel that they are the victims of a dastardly persecution and, making public protest, end as the occupants of mental hospitals. Occasionally they do not progress as far as this, but become tramps and prostitutes and fall into the hands of the law by some petty theft or misdemeanour. Often it is at this stage when they draw attention to themselves that they are examined by the psychologist and their whole unhappy history comes to light. These are the children who have been called " constitutional psychopaths ", a bad name which suggests that their condition is hereditary, whereas it is but the product of environment.

Another rather sad type is the child who is regarded as a mental defective and treated accordingly all its life. This child nearly always has lived in an atmosphere which has been emotionally painful to it and has never been allowed to develop emotionally, with the consequence that its intellect has never been able to show itself as it really is. This child passes through school slowly and is regarded as a dull and stupid child, and when it leaves it is usually thrust into a manual or domestic post which it hates but is often unable to alter. It is fortunate for such a child to develop a neurosis and fall into the hands of a psychologist who, in treating the neurosis, may be able to release its retarded intellectual powers. The writer has had such a case under his care—this was a girl who had been regarded as extremely stupid when she was a child. She had, however, been treated very unkindly by her father and mother. The father's ill-treatment of her brother eventually led to his imprisonment. She did badly at school and when she left school was able to obtain employment only as a nursemaid. She hated this and developed a nervous illness which led her into the writer's care. She was treated, with the result that she not only lost her illness, but when she had an intelligence test performed it showed that she was the possessor of an intellect equal to that of a university professor. Since treatment she has been able to obtain a post of secretary, which was more suited to her mentality, and has been much happier. It is very necessary with such cases as this that an intelligence test should be performed. They are most deceptive and the impression of stupidity is a very real one.

Much has been written about the personality of the epileptic and the suggestion has come from America that one should be able to diagnose the epileptic before the onset of fits. It has been said that the epileptic is self-centred and egotistical. That he always displays an excess of religiosity in his behaviour. He covers his selfishness and self-interest under a cloak of apparent benevolence, and although he appears to be considerate to others he is in reality very uninterested in them. All this may be true but, in the writer's opinion, it is not sufficiently definite for one to be certain that a child who shows these characteristics is necessarily a potential epileptic. Children who show these characteristics may be showing some defect in their personalities, but one would be bold to insist that these personality defects will lead inevitably to epilepsy.

Again, it is unusual to find any evidence of depressive illnesses in children. Many writers have suggested that the melancholic often shows himself to be a sad miserable person long before he develops a true mental illness. It is very unusual to find prolonged depressions in children before puberty, although at puberty one sometimes finds children who feel sad but do not know why they do so. If such children come from a family where their parents have suffered from depression, then it is a danger sign and every effort should be made to adjust the child and to remove the beginnings of this type of reaction.

A curious reaction which is to be regarded rather as a danger signal than as a personality aberration is what may be called " acting fantasies ". This shows an inability to distinguish between reality and fantasy. It is, of course, quite normal for a small child to find some difficulty in distinguishing between the real and the fantastic. A child of four will tell one that a huge lion chased it down the street, and it would be quite right and proper for the adult to join in the fantasy by some such remark as : " Couldn't you manage to kill it ? " or " Perhaps that was the one which chased me last week." In other children when such a trait is to be found it is to be regarded as abnormal. The child who boasts that his father has enormous estates in Roumania and owns four Rolls-Royce cars, and so on, is probably suffering from pathological lying. If this is allowed to develop without treating the cause it is probable that the child will grow into a thoroughly unreliable person or (since one tends to put one's fantasies into reality) will one day impersonate a duke and involve himself in hotel expenses which he cannot pay. A large number of criminals start in this way, and even if they are brought up against reality with a sudden jolt they have too often lost their reputations and been branded as habitual criminals before it happens.

The descriptions which have been given are somewhat arbitrary and artificial. This is because the various types of reaction are not found in a state of nature in an isolated condition but are naturally mixed to some extent. For example the shy, withdrawn child usually shows some timidity and may to a certain extent display the characteristics of the over-conscientious child. These are compatible reactions and naturally occur together if the environment is suitable to produce them. Again, the over-aggressive child may show some of the characteristics of the obstinate mulish child and so on. Naturally incompatible reactions such as shyness and over-aggressiveness cannot occur at the same time in the same child. This does not really invalidate the description of a personality deviation as a persistent reaction because the compatible reactions are all more or less of the same type.

It might be of interest to discuss the treatment of these conditions since a certain amount can be corrected by the parent or teacher. We have seen in the discussion of personality deviations that they are caused by a number of conditions. Firstly by the defects in the parents upon whom the child models itself, and later in the environment to which the child has to adjust itself. It is impossible for the parents to correct themselves, but those who intend to marry and have children would be wise to have treatment for their own nervous illnesses before they do so. Those who are already married, if they are the unfortunate victims of nervous or mental illness would be wise to have treatment before their illness affects their children. If all those who have felt dissatisfaction in their own personalities were to have treatment before they had children they would feel less dissatisfaction in the personalities of their children when they watch them growing up. The other factor in the prevention of personality defects is to allow the child to enjoy the widest possible contacts and not over-protect it. One frequently finds in only children (who are very precious to their parents), and in children who come from a family where a child has been lost through an accident, that they are not allowed to mix freely with other children. They are so over-sheltered that they have never to react to any than perfectly familiar surroundings. These children cannot possibly develop such healthy responses as the child who plays, fights and works with his equals and bears blows and buffets as often as he gives them.

Although it is most desirable to prevent the development of personality disorders, it is even more essential to prevent their growth when they have already appeared, and this can only be done by attacking the cause. All psychological treatment of children must inevitably fall into two categories. Firstly, the alteration of the child's environment in order that it can respond correctly to its new conditions ; and secondly, the alteration of the child by the direct attack of psychotherapy by more or less analytical methods. To alter the child's environment is easy and inexpensive, while to treat it analytically is prolonged and expensive. Nevertheless, it must be remembered that to change the environment does not produce a permanent change for a long while, and if the environment reverts to its previous level the child is likely to drop back into its old reactions. Psychotherapy is more likely to produce such permanent change in the child that it is able to face even the causal environment with impunity.

When one attempts to manipulate a child's surroundings one can either add to them or subtract from them. Often the mere addition to the environment will suffice for remarkable improvement. The addition should always be in the direction which adds new reactions to the child's experience and allows it to develop in some way. For example, a shy, withdrawn child will often respond marvellously when it is taken from the home where it feels cramped and introduced to such a new environment as is provided by the Boy Scouts or a boys' club. Once out of contact with the factors which have produced its shyness the child will often open out surprisingly after a while, mix freely with its equals, and be less fearful with its superiors. Often a boy who lives in a completely feminine atmosphere provided by his widowed mother and sisters will alter considerably with such a change of environment.

The subtraction from the environment of undesirable elements makes it necessary that one studies the child's surroundings very carefully. One must discover what factor is causing its illness and eliminate it. Sometimes it is a bullying brother or a drunken father and so on, sometimes a doting mother who hampers its every movement with her mistaken attitude to it. It is by no means easy always to discover the cause and, even when it is discovered, to eliminate it. Often one can localize the cause by the fact that the child behaves in a differential manner—that it is open and frank at home while it is obstinate and surly at school. Such a situation points to the factor being in the school and the behaviour of the teacher may be found to be at fault. It is better to alter the environment by persuading the teacher where he is at fault than to move the child to another school (which may give it the impression that difficulties are to be avoided rather than faced squarely).

As an example of the excellent results which can be obtained by removing the causal factor and substituting some better environment is shown by the case of a boy aged ten who was suffering from stammering. It was discovered in investigating the case that the boy's father came home drunk every night and knocked the boy about in his drunken rages. Fortunately before one could draw the mother's attention to the fact that the father's behaviour was making her son ill, she had decided herself that she could stand it no longer. She and her son left the father and went to live elsewhere. The boy was recommended to join a boys' club and did so. His stammer disappeared as if by magic and he appeared perfectly well. Not until he saw his father in the street and dreamed about his previous experience did he start stammering again. When he had been able to talk about this his stammer disappeared and never returned. This example shows clearly that the father was the causal factor and not until he was eliminated did the child find it possible to react normally to his surroundings.

The manipulation of the environment and the removal of the cause of the child's aberration can often be done by the parent or teacher once the kind of situation is known and much rough and ready psychotherapy can be performed in this way with excellent results. When, however, the child does not respond to alterations in his surroundings and still shows the same type of reaction in spite of the most favourable conditions, it may be necessary that more meticulous treatment should be applied. This must inevitably take the form of some type of analytical treatment, and is not suitable for the use of the teacher or parent.

A good example of such treatment is shown by the case of a boy aged seven who was self-absorbed, timid and shy. He did not play games, and spoke with a stammer. It was discovered that the boy's elder brother was the parents' favourite. They were told that they must suppress their tendency to favouritism and treat the brothers equally. They did so, but even this did not produce much change in the younger child. It was then found possible to penetrate the boy's shyness by getting him to draw and interpret pictures. By simple analytical methods one was able to release his pent-up emotion. The result was that the patient lost his stammer and the relations between the brothers were greatly improved. They now played happily together and the former stammerer rose rapidly from 27th place to 3rd place in class. His whole personality changed and he was able to be much more frank, open and self-confident.

In this short account an attempt has been made to show the structure of the personality and how such a structure can be formed from the parents and the environment, how disease processes occur and how they may be observed, how treated and eliminated.

It has been said that there are no abnormal children—only abnormal parents. This is exaggerated and unpalatable, but, nevertheless, there is no doubt that the faults in the parents' personalities are mirrored in their children. It follows therefore that every child we allow to grow up with some gross defect in its personality carries with it the potentiality of being a parent who will continue a fault which may do infinite damage to our civilization. If this is a depressing thought, we can console ourselves by the fact that every time we correct a defect in a child we are not treating that child alone, but an infinite number of children yet unborn.

V. HABITS

By PATERSON BROWN, M.B., CH.B., D.P.M.,
MEDICAL DIRECTOR, NORTH WESTERN LONDON
CHILD GUIDANCE CLINIC

V. HABITS

BY PATERSON BROWN, M.B., CH.B., D.P.M.,
MEDICAL DIRECTOR, NORTH WESTERN LONDON CHILD
GUIDANCE CLINIC

HABITS make the man, or so it is said. The thought of certain habits strikes terror in many a parent's heart; and while some parents are less disturbed than others, all tend to take habits seriously, particularly in childhood, where we feel, and quite rightly, that they have their origin. Habits may be good or bad, but in this chapter, while the general factors operative in the production of habits will be discussed, emphasis will be laid on those factors connected with the formation of *bad* habits, and ways in which they may be avoided or relieved.

Habit is the name given to any form of conduct which is repetitive, but usually only when it has become exaggerated or departs in some way from what we are accustomed to regard as normal. Habits exist in perplexing variety, and probably no one is free from them in some form. It may be helpful to note some of the more usual habits and see if we can detect some common characteristics which will help us to understand them.

Thumb-sucking, nail-biting, masturbation, body-

149

rocking, head-banging, grimacing, pulling the hair, rubbing the nose or ear, sucking the sheet or placing objects in the mouth, hoarding rubbish, dirty ways, laziness and constipation ; these are all common, and yet the list could be doubled or trebled without difficulty.

The first fact which excites comment is the great frequency with which particular parts of the body are involved. We also notice that it is very often not so much a particular part of the body, as some function associated with that part, which has become exaggerated and detached from its original purpose. The simplest example of this is to be found in activities concerned with the mouth, which include sucking, placing objects in the mouth, and nail-biting. Indeed, we could isolate the particular function of sucking, as the number of objects which may be sucked is legion. The problem which requires explanation is why particular or, if we think in terms of the body, local functions should become so developed as to appear purposeless. The answer is the same as is found in general medicine, where we are accustomed to regard a local increase of tissue or of function as the result of some increased demand. That is why the muscles increase with exercise or hard physical labour, or why the heart may enlarge in response to some impediment to the circulation, as in high blood pressure.

Let us consider again the question of sucking, and thumb-sucking in particular, because this early act is, of course, a normal phenomenon which we cannot imagine the infant without.

Thumb-sucking may, however, become exaggerated in response to some difficulty associated with the process. The difficulty may arise externally, as when the child is insufficiently fed or the mother has nipples which are cracked or turned inwards, but it may equally lie within the child itself. An example would be if the child has a heavy cold, so that it cannot breathe and suck at the same time, or if it has a cleft palate, which is an absence of the roof of the mouth and which may obviously disturb the process of sucking. In circumstances such as these we may expect exaggerations of this early and universal activity.

There is, however, another possibility which we can again illustrate from general medicine. The local exaggeration may be a response to difficulties in some other region. The heart, which enlarges in response to increased blood pressure, may be reacting ultimately to disease in the kidneys, the ill-effects of which can only be overcome by increased pressure in the circulation, which assists them in their task of filtration.

To take other, perhaps simpler, examples, a man with one arm will have that arm more developed than if he had two, and the blind man develops his powers of touch and hearing to a degree which surprises the normal-sighted person. These mechanisms, then, are compensatory, and we find them at work in the formation of habits. When sucking becomes exaggerated, it is to compensate for difficulties elsewhere. The child may be unhappy for many reasons unconnected with feeding—perhaps because of bright lights, loud

noises or some discomfort associated with its body—
and these may all contribute to the exaggeration of
the sucking habit. These environmental causes,
which are external to the " me " of the child, can
be very numerous, particularly in later years, and
even in adult life.

Not very long ago I saw a woman with a very
curious habit, or rather, in this case, a compulsion.
She could not bear her hands to be idle if she was
quietly talking to someone or reading a book.
The result of this anxiety was that knitting had
become for her a necessity in these circumstances.
The reason for this was very interesting. Her
husband was a peculiar, abnormal person, and, in
her own words : " If I didn't keep my hands busy
I would murder him." This instance is illuminating
because the cause of the habit is so clearly revealed
as well as its purposefulness. Knitting is obviously
a very much better solution for her anxiety than
to murder her husband. Another way in which the
process might be expressed would be to say that
an aggressive destructive impulse had been turned
from its original goal to one which was socially
useful.

This case, however, is unusual, and we recognize
that many children develop habits without suffering
any such anxiety-provoking situations. The puzzle
is solved when we discover that children can and
do suffer from anxieties which are just as acute as
those for which there is real external cause, without
there being any disturbance of importance in the
environment. The reason for this lies in the
nature of the mind itself, which we shall have to

review in some detail if we are to grasp the manner in which these anxieties arise, and learn how habits are developed in the course of finding relief. All this may become more credible if we remember the frequency, and indeed normality, of irrational fears in childhood. Who does not know of the child who is afraid of one of the following : of the dark, of insects, of small animals such as mice, large animals like horses, of being alone, of being in company, of going to the lavatory alone or attended, of open or enclosed spaces, of nakedness or of particular garments, of masks, heights, noises, and thunder or lightning ?

Let me tell you of another case which illustrates much of what has been discussed. A boy of nine had contracted the habit of blinking his eyes. He did not have the habit when I saw him first, but he did have a great fear of any long object being pointed in the direction of his eyes, and if this was done he flinched and looked away. With the development of the habit of blinking, however, the fear disappeared. I saw him still later, and this time he was wearing glasses for a visual defect, and in turn the blinking had disappeared. The defensive value of the habit is obvious. It defended the boy against a fear which was present in his mind; at the same time it is doubtful if the habit would have developed but for the coincident visual defect. This was the local cause, otherwise why should the blinking have disappeared when he took to glasses ?

Let us summarize the argument up to this point, and then proceed to examine this new factor peculiar to the nature of mind itself. A habit appears to be a local exaggeration of function, and there are three causes for this.

Firstly, the habit may be the result of an increased local need, just as grit in the eye may cause blinking, or a cold cause coughing. Secondly, it may compensate for some painful condition in the environment, or in the child, but if so one which the child himself feels to be external.

Finally, the nature of mind is such that acute anxieties may arise and have to be dealt with in the presence of circumstances which appear to be innocuous. The boy who flinched at long objects knew that they were harmless and that his reaction was due to a misjudgment. The difficulty lay in his own mind, and can only be explained when we understand better what goes on in the mind.

It would appear that the mind operates in a condition of tension, which is a result of the need to satisfy the instincts. Together with those instincts which minister to the needs and desires of the individual, are the instincts which remove obstructions and dangers, and if these instincts fail to achieve their object the tension within the mind is increased, and may be felt as *anxiety*. Mental growth is very largely concerned with the progressively developed capacity either to bear or to relieve the tension engendered by the instincts.

The reasons why anxiety is so acute in the young child are many. One factor is the relative helplessness or dependence of the small child upon its environment. There can be no doubt that the child may feel this situation very acutely. Anyone who knows children has observed the pleasure with which they will stand on a chair or other object and proudly declare they are taller than you are. In its play the child's powers are in marked contrast to its capacities in real life. Toys are treated as living people, and power of life and death is held over them. Moreover, it is a simple matter to bring the dead back to life, to make them accomplish impossible feats, or to endow them with magical powers. This is all enormously reassuring to the child. The child who can play in this way will not feel like the man to whom only one talent had been vouchsafed, and who was therefore altogether too poor and needy for any adventuring in the world.

One factor, then, is the relative helplessness and dependence of the young child. Another is that, apart from anything else, the child is subject to very intense feelings, which may be partly a result of the necessary limitations to its actions. We are apt to forget that what may be an intellectual conception of convenience or æsthetics to the adult, is to the child a simple and intense instance of good and bad. I remember a mother who both in theory and practice allowed her child every liberty. At the same time she clearly valued cleanliness and good manners, but never insisted on them and never expressed to her child that there was anything particularly bad about their absence. Nevertheless, she was surprised one day to find her child in hysterical distress over a drop of urine which had fallen accidentally while the child was in the lavatory. The reason for this distress was that the child's inner mental world of extreme conceptions had been influenced by the mother's unconscious example. What to the mother was merely nice, to the child was essential.

While recognizing the intensity of the feelings in the child's mind, we must not forget that it is also very concrete in its thought. Once a child who came to see me picked an apple in the garden, then looked at me with a glance of enquiry, and said, " If you liked apples like I do you wouldn't let me have any, would you ? " With the child it is a case of all or nothing, and an object or a course of action is for the moment either wholly good or wholly bad.

If we can accept the existence of acute anxieties in the child's mind, and the foregoing argument as giving some of the reasons for this conclusion, let us go on to consider some of the methods by which relief from anxiety is obtained. We shall discover that these methods are very intimately bound up with habit formation.

Limits of space make it impossible to describe more than a few of the known mechanisms, but all of the following are frequent. They can be called (a) adventuring, (b) finding or pursuing pleasure, (c) seeking pain or self-punishment or renunciation, and (d) restitution or restoration. We must remember, throughout, that all these processes may be unconscious, just as the instinctual aim may be unconscious, and even the anxiety itself may not be felt while it is being dispersed in some form of conduct.

The first " mechanism " of adventuring, or

reality-testing as it is sometimes called, works as if the child put to itself the question : " Is the world really as bad as I imagine it to be, and dare I risk finding out ? " It is an exploratory gesture and is one of the mechanisms involved when children are flouting danger. The child feels its anxieties must be set at rest, that its fears must be proved groundless. Perhaps the child is unsafe in traffic, or on a bicycle, or cannot be left alone in the house because of a tendency to play with fire, or cannot be left in the garden because it will climb to dangerous positions and be in danger of falling. In all these cases the child, while apparently without any sense of danger, is really pursued by a fear which it must deny or refute. It is the same with children who eat peculiar objects, or place dirty things in their mouth, or perhaps destroy their clothes. As evidence of this you will find that it is most often the parent who is anxious lest the child should do certain things which has the child who does them. The reason is that parents' fears, however expressed, increase those of their children, so that the reality-testing mechanism comes into operation. We often hear it said to a child who has some habit or other : " If you do that no one will like you " ; now we see how such a " warning " will only increase the child's insecurity, and make the habit all the more necessary. In just the same way threats, whatever their nature, often have an effect which is the opposite to that intended. The child who is threatened with the policeman may not *feel* an increased amount of anxiety, but the presence of anxiety may be shown by the child becoming more cheeky and perhaps defying the policeman, or even making friends with him.

Pleasure-seeking is an activity which almost describes itself. It is an attempt to turn a situation to advantage, to extract from it any pleasure which may be available and which will offset anxiety. Two examples occur to me. The first was a little girl of nine. She was on bad terms with her father and mother, even to the extent of saying to her mother, " Shut up, you." She was constantly putting herself into danger, and one day she succeeded in gassing herself during her mother's absence from the house for a few minutes. When her mother returned she found the house full of gas, which she quickly dispersed, but the child remained unconscious for three-quarters of an hour. One would expect her to have been frightened and cowed by such an experience, but it thrilled her and she derived further pleasure from it by boasting about it to strangers, thus creating a minor sensation. There was also some pleasure to be obtained from frightening her mother.

The other case is of an older child, a girl aged fourteen. I saw her because she was surly and rude at home. She happened to have a bent back, and her mother thought it remarkable that she enjoyed showing herself to doctors and medical students. Yet the reason is plain enough, for when showing her back she felt important; the situation became enjoyable and painful feelings were reduced.

These are extreme cases, but illustrate how it is just where the spots are sensitive that the ointment of pleasure is most necessary. The trouble is that adults are apt to take a child's pleasure rather seriously and interfere with it, although it may be serving a useful purpose. In a sentence, pleasure is pain-relieving, and it is one of nature's ways of making life tolerable.

The same mechanism is found very widely distributed in the case of habits. There is usually a deeper painful situation behind each exaggeration. This has already been explained in the case of thumb-sucking. It applies equally to all those habits connected with manipulations of the body— rubbing the nose or eye, picking the nose, or placing a finger in the ear, and masturbation, or the evocation of pleasant sensations from the genitals. It is interesting also to see how one habit may replace another. We have thumb-sucking in the infant, placing objects in the mouth in the child, and smoking in the adult. I have seen cases where excessive masturbation has resulted from the rigid suppression of thumb-sucking, and, in the older child, where it is helping it to escape from a sense of failure at school or rebelliousness against authority. Not infrequently to forbid a habit is to encourage a condition which is worse.

It is a common practice to measure one's worth in terms of one's possessions, and so pleasure-seeking may also take the form of collecting. If anxiety is very great, bad habits may be the result. This is the case when all the child's efforts are concentrated on what he can get out of people, and when his possessions are jealously guarded as a sole source of pleasure. Miserly habits are not infrequent in childhood. When anxiety is not so great there is pleasure in sharing one's possessions with others, because the fear of being robbed is less urgent. This applies not only to articles, which may be enthusiastically collected, but also to less material possessions such as knowledge, or prowess at sport, or the ability to pass examinations.

The third mechanism, that of pain-seeking or self-punishment, is both the most important mechanism and the most difficult one to understand. Self-punishment is in a sense an inward testing of reality. It is a reflection inwards of feelings of hostility which were originally directed outwards. It is no good looking at another person and thinking : " I wish I could kill you " (cf. the phrase " if looks could kill "), if that other person is either more powerful or necessary to our existence in some way than we are. In that case we will fear him, thinking that he must be feeling similar hostility towards us, and the only way out is to bring the feared retaliation upon ourselves in our need to allay the anxiety aroused by our destructive impulses. A small boy I know saw a lady some distance away whom he called an alligator. A little later, rushing past her, he slipped and hurt his knee. It was no accident that he was hurt, and not the " alligator ", whom he feared, because of his own aggressive feelings. It is a puzzle to many people why some children are so prone to accidents or unfortunate happenings, and this is the reason. It is very often the result of hostile feelings for which there is no direct outlet, as in the above instance. Some children are always losing toys, or dirtying and destroying their clothes, or losing friends, and as a rule the above mechanism is responsible for these events.

Most mechanisms, however, are mixed; nail-biting is a very clear example of this. The pleasure of biting is indulged in, but there is a hostile element involved which is directed against the self. Moreover, the original hostility may still achieve some direct satisfaction through the annoyance which the habit gives to others, and equally some additional pleasure may be extracted from the general interest aroused, whilst all the time fears are being set at rest by the discovery that the condition is relatively harmless. Habits, however, are not always harmless, and this illustrates the force which is sometimes present behind these expressions of instinct. I have seen a child of seven who could not be stopped from swallowing pins and needles, and who had in consequence already undergone three major operations. It was impossible to dress another child in any kind of woollen garment, as the child always unpicked the wool and ate it. These markedly abnormal appetites are, of course, unusual, but in a minor degree they are frequently encountered among normal people.

Renunciation is an extension of the mechanism along another direction. Some children are so afraid of their aggressive or possessive wishes that they have to go without things. They may even go without food or refuse sweets. More usual examples are the refusal to eat certain types of food, such as meat or vegetables.

Other children may have to give their toys or their money away, and, perversely as it would seem, take pleasure in being without possessions or friends.

Self-punishment is neither a purely passive mechanism nor a purely destructive one, for it is often very largely instrumental in restoring good relations after they have been strained by feelings of hostility.

Restitution, the last mechanism of all, is a way of escape from self-punishment. In it, our efforts are bent towards restoring or helping the person whom we have attacked in our imagination. It derives its energy from a double source. In the first place, the person may be loved as well as hated, and, secondly, any fear we may have of being attacked by them is set at rest.

Behaviour becomes compulsive and repetitive when the mechanism is not succeeding, so that it is a cause of habits, as well as a method whereby they become unnecessary. The child who gives its toys away, or who is easily led, may be making compulsive restitution to the other person, very often as a means of dominating him, perhaps by becoming necessary to him, or in order to remain as a critic. This satisfies destructive as well as constructive impulses, and the process requires indefinite repetition. What we can remember is that the older child may find it helpful to assist its parents in some way, or to tidy up where it has made a mess, or to give a present, and we must not discourage these activities. This is one of the chief ways in which good habits are formed.

Now that we have some appreciation of how habits are formed during the often obscure workings of the mind, we can take up the general question of how we should treat a child with habits which have become excessive. By now we realize that it is not the habit which we treat, but the child. It is not the symptom that requires attack, but the underlying anxiety. If the child masturbates (pleasure-seeking) or bites its nails (self-punishment), or has no sense of danger or responsibility (reality-testing), then we will not interfere with these activities in any direct way, but ask ourselves first if there is some local stimulus, and secondly, if the environment is reassuring.

It must be remembered that any direct challenging of the habit will either increase its necessity in one form or another or spoil the child's disposition.

The local causes for various habits are as numerous as the habits themselves, but they are not that which gives the habit its very dynamic quality. Touching the ear may originally be associated with some irritation or inflammation in the passage; picking the nose may be a sequel to catarrh; a persistent cough follows a sore throat; and blinking a visual defect or grit in the eye. One of the examples which is most frequently given is that of masturbation as a sequel to irritation in or about the genitals. Naturally our first care will be the relief of the local condition, but what we must not forget is that no matter how potent the local stimulus may be, the habit would not persist had it not become a channel for the relief of anxiety. Some of the most troublesome habits to treat are those connected with speaking, whether pronunciation, tone of voice, or word production, as in lisping or stammering. One of the reasons for this difficulty is that so much attention is concentrated on the symptom itself, rather than upon the underlying causes. Very frequently the parent will seek for some surgeon, who will operate on the child's throat, hoping that relief will be obtained in this way. What is forgotten is the purposefulness of the habit, and the fact that many habits are in fact the sequel to an operation with all the disturbance this means in the child's mind. I saw a boy of ten with a very severe and constant blinking of the eyes, and this had followed directly on an operation for circumcision at the age of seven. Such cases are by no means rare.

The next point that arises is whether there are internal difficulties which can be relieved. Is the child in generally good health? Is it enjoying school and meeting with a fair measure of success? Comparisons between children are usually invidious. A child will find it much less wounding to live in an atmosphere of indifference than one where another child is openly preferred, perhaps because he is more successful or fits in better with the parents' idea of what he should be like. Just as one child may proceed from success to success, another may go from bad to worse, for this very reason. Too much driving of any kind will be bad, whatever form it may take, or whatever the motive. Often it is some added responsibility, such as the stress of scholarship examinations, which will be the final straw leading to breakdown. Some parents may concentrate more particularly on sports, and this will have the same bad effect on the child if he is less strong, or less interested in sport than in other activities. Every child has its individuality, which must be allowed for.

Then there are the subtler forms of parental anxiety, of which the parent may be unaware, but which surely add to the burden on the child. There are first those parents who do too much for their children. Perhaps without realizing it, they are full of fear that the child cannot do anything without them. Without knowing it they lack confidence in the child and increase its fears. In the first place, it may be the parent rather than the child who fears it cannot pass an examination, choose its friends, eat a good meal if unwatched, or generally fend for itself. Another reason why doing too much is so bad for the child is that the child is deprived of the reassuring pleasure which comes from finding it can do things it may be in doubt about. If I should see, say, a mother and child in consultation, it is usual rather than exceptional for the mother at the end of the interview to turn to the child and say, "Now, say good-bye to the doctor," without giving the child choice or opportunity in the matter of doing so for itself. The child that cannot leave its mother is very often the child of a mother that cannot leave it. We can judge a situation better by the results of what we do than by our feelings about it. The mother of a fine healthy boy of ten was very unhappy about his poor appetite, and in spite of his obvious health and the fact that she continued to buy him

Jersey milk " as he needs the extra nourishment ", assured me very emphatically that she did not really worry about him. I do believe the boy is difficult at meals, but I should ascribe the trouble to his mother's anxiety, even although she is unaware of its existence. Actually the atmosphere created is more important than the things done, and this makes it difficult to give advice. We may unconsciously be afraid of our children, and keep them at too great a distance, ultimately producing the same reaction as if we were to do too much. The child may lack the help and encouragement which it would derive from our spontaneous pleasure in what it does and, further, will feel our uncertainty, which may make it feel uncertain in return. Some parents may take too modest a view of their children's attainments, and others too glorified a view.

Most unfortunately, reason alone, just when we expect most help from it, proves of little avail. If our feelings are wrong, we shall tend to do the wrong thing. I remember very vividly a small boy of seven who stammered. He was brought up by very cultured parents. They did not encourage warlike and blood-thirsty games. There were no soldiers or guns in his nursery and, further, he was taught kindness to animals to such a degree that slugs in the garden were protected rather than killed. To his parents' intense astonishment, they were told that, in the first ten minutes with me, he let off the greatest flood of cruel fantasy I have ever heard, of cutting, of killing and of torturing in every imaginable way. These feelings may not be reasonable, but they are part of our heritage, a heritage we shall gradually grow out of if they are not suppressed. If they are, some habit in which self-punishment predominates is likely.

Reasoning with the child neglects the intense feeling-life of the child, and this must not be denied outlet, since it places too much responsibility on the child's shoulders, rather than removing it. Giving reasons to the child for our requests is different. This is useful, and helpful if it is not too much a necessity on our part to placate the child. In the latter event it will sense our fear, and react as before. Another common way in which over-anxiety in the parent is revealed even when not felt is by an exaggerated calmness or deliberateness which is no more normal than over-emotionalism. A parent may be ever on the alert not to show any strong feelings to the child under the mistaken impression that it is being saved from some harmful experience. A special case of this is never letting the child see that one is angry or annoyed. We are only bottling up the emotion, which will assume some more disguised and therefore sinister form, and coincidently the child will develop a greater fear of its own strong feelings when they are so rare in others, and apparently so to be avoided.

The fear on the part of the parent of strong feelings in the child is often seen in the proud reference to the fact that their children show no jealousy of each other. This is not always a matter for congratulation. The jealousy may be suppressed, increasing the tensions in the mind.

This results from the child sensing that this is the reaction which the parent hopes for, and perhaps prepares for by means of explanations regarding the expected arrival of a brother or sister. I do not mean explanations are bad; on the contrary; but underlying the explanation there is often the hope that danger has been averted, and the future is up to the child. It is as if the parent said to the child, " I've done my bit, now you do yours."

Enough has been said of difficult environmental situations. It is more important to realize that a few habits or a few symptoms of discord are normal in the developing child, and represent points where anxieties are whirling up like eddies in a tide. It is only when either the child or the external situation is abnormal that the habit is likely to become severe or persistent.

The next thing is to discuss ways in which the child can be helped, apart from expert treatment, after everything possible has been done to remove any external impediment or difficulty. All that can be said follows from what has been written already, but it may be summarized in the form of a few principles. Control the child and prevent excesses, but allow the maximum possible freedom of expression to its primitive feelings and actions of aggression. In other words, let it be somewhat rough and dirty without let or hindrance, and make the minimum number of demands for adult standards of conduct. All the time one must be ready to help him, but not to do everything he dictates.

Before closing this chapter, let us sum up and discuss some particular habits in detail. We know

now that habits like most symptoms may mean almost anything, or nothing. Each case must be judged on its merits, the criterion being the general development of the personality. Habits do not often result from single incidents, but more frequently from repeated small incidents, which have a cumulative effect in increasing anxiety. They may arise at any age, but are certainly commonest during the years we are interested in. To determine their full meaning we should have to go back to the time of their origin, and then further back to the reason for the excessive anxieties in the mind, and in addition there is the reason in the present which may be responsible for its continuance. Picking the nose may be a form of erotic indulgence following on a cold, but its continuance may depend on the attention it attracts or the tension following upon the threat that " if you do that no one will like you ".

Probably the largest and most troublesome class of habits are those affecting daily routine activities. For instance, difficulties over getting up or going to bed, personal needs such as washing, dressing or undressing, having the hair combed or cut, or general carelessness and untidiness, or positively irritating behaviour as when doors are banged or left open, lights left on, and so on. All of these are usually connected with unconscious fears. One boy of ten I know had either to be dressed by his mother, or entirely by himself, and if some dispute arose he complained of feeling " gritty ", and the process of dressing had to be repeated anew from the beginning, to his mother's infinite annoyance.

Some children feel when their clothes are taken off
that they are losing some possession or being
exposed to attack. Others object to putting
clothes on because they feel bound and unconsciously fear the restriction. I have known several
children who in going to the lavatory had conscious
fears either of being attacked or robbed. One, a
child of seven, was afraid to go to the lavatory
because he feared that when he pulled the plug an
animal would spring out from an adjoining room
and eat him up. These fears are irrational, of
course, and the result of anxiety deep in the child's
mind. Perhaps more than anything else they are a
reflection of the child's own hostility and aggression
along the lines already explained. When difficulty
is made over going to bed, the child may be afraid
of dying during the night, and when the night is
over it may fear getting up, because of the tasks of
the day, which he fears he may be unable to accomplish. Both ideas are often present at the same
time. Some of the habits still bear trace of the
original hostility which is felt towards the adult,
as, for instance, the banging of doors. Bed-wetting
is particularly troublesome with some children.
Some kind of physical weakness may perhaps be
partly responsible for the habit, but it is probable
that it would not occur in the absence of excessive
anxiety. It is again the result of most mechanisms
in varying proportions. That pleasure and reassurance can be derived from bed-wetting seems
scarcely credible, but cases are not rare where these
factors are fully conscious, and in addition some
hostility can be presumed from the nature of

the trouble itself. Unfortunately, only too often measures adopted for its relief are more likely to lead to its continuance. Frequent rousings which interrupt sleep result in a feeling of resentment, or the wetting will be used as a means of dominating the person who rouses the child. When fluids are restricted, so are the child's pleasures in life. Many children have been cured by the removal of all restrictions and precautions, which is contrary to the advice usually given, but is psychologically very sound. Punishment is usually worse than useless. Always when we are dealing with a person with a troublesome habit let us proceed with forbearance, noting that the person is only too often shy and shut-in, or noisy and rebellious, to an abnormal degree. This is not only to be associated with the cause of the habit, but also with its unwise treatment. Nowhere is this more true than in the habit of masturbation, and we can foresee the dangers which cannot be separated from indignant punishment or condemnation. Genuine reassurance is more likely than anything else to do good, but it is sometimes wise to ignore the habit if it is not severe.

In conclusion, I should like to say a few words about some difficulties which cropped up during a very small part of the treatment of a boy of fifteen. These difficulties might have occurred as individual habits in childhood with little disadvantage to the boy, but they accumulated under the surface and serious mental illness was the result. First, with regard to food he alternated between excessive greediness, which made him feel guilty, and eating

practically nothing for days.   Eating he referred to
as temptation and giving in.   Sleep was similarly
feared and avoided, and he would be awake for
nights on end.   In bed he had a fear he was dead,
and that his heart was not beating, or that he could
not stand up to an unknown assailant.   Then he
felt he had to keep his eyes open all night.   Coming
to see me represented a challenge to look in my
eyes which he could not meet.   This was succeeded
by a phase of closing his eyes when anxiety about
the thought of attacking me became great.   To do
any of these self-forbidden acts was his greatest
triumph.   During this period he said he had been
doing a lot of reading and staring ; in other words,
of taking things in with his eyes ; and a further
development was a fantasy that a Véry light bullet
was not only lighting up darkness in a war, but
entering his stomach so that he died in agony.
This is an interesting link between the fear of
eating and looking and of sleeping.   The sadistic
or hostile aspect of these ideas came out in further
fantasies that he would tear my eyes out, that my
eyes were blue and so was ice, and that he was
treading on thin ice.   Then he said that even when
the sky was blue a torrent might come down ;
this provided a link with his fear of urinating
destructively.   He had, as a matter of fact, wet the
bed at one time, which is a further reason why he
was afraid of bed and darkness.   You will not be
surprised to hear that he was also afraid to go to
the lavatory, yet going to the lavatory was also
associated with various excesses.

These are indeed tangled events and again strain

credulity, but they are fantasies which may be dominating a person without their awareness. It is much better that they should achieve minimal but frequent expression in ordinary everyday doings, rather than become a source of illness. Let me say it again; be tolerant of habits, and you will often be saved from worse disasters. Habits make the man. They also save the man from an undesirable accumulation of anxiety.

VI. NEUROSIS IN SCHOOL-CHILDREN

By C. L. C. BURNS, M.R.C.S., L.R.C.P., D.P.M.,
DIRECTOR, BIRMINGHAM CHILD GUIDANCE CLINIC

VI. NEUROSIS IN SCHOOL-CHILDREN

BY C. L. C. BURNS, M.R.C.S., L.R.C.P., D.P.M., DIRECTOR,
BIRMINGHAM CHILD GUIDANCE CLINIC

IN a lecture·on nervous children given to a parent-teacher association, the parents were asked to say whether they could lay claim to children who suffered from " nerves " and if so what were their complaints. About 20 per cent of the parents held up their hands, and the list of symptoms included timidity and fears, twitching, stammering, night fears, insomnia, and lack of confidence.

This indicates first of all that nervous children of school age are not uncommon, and secondly that the net which includes this popular category is a wide one. A further investigation would reveal a more comprehensive list and would be found to include such traits as excessive shyness, unsociability and dreaminess—states of mind which are often grouped under the term " personality disorders ".

Again, when we come to consider those complaints which are described as " behaviour disorders ", such as tempers, destructiveness, rebellion to authority and delinquency, we shall find that these children too will generally show signs of " nerves ". The defiant young gangster of the streets may be afraid of the dark.

Since questions involving character or person-

ality and habit are dealt with in other chapters,
the scope of the discussion in this chapter must be
confined mainly to a consideration of "*nervous
children*" of school age—those children who show
the kind of symptoms which any intelligent teacher
or parent would describe as coming within this
vague yet fairly circumscribed category. They
would correspond in the main to the group of
"*neuroses*" which Professor Burt has recently described as the "Asthenic" or weak, as contrasted with
the "Sthenic" or strong—the latter being applied to
such reactions as anger and aggression generally.

Now a neurosis of any kind involves both an
attitude or state of mind, and an action, or series of
actions ; it is both feeling and action. The nervous
child is in a state of fear or, to use a more technical
term, anxiety, but this may be outwardly shown not
only by his expression and demeanour towards
others but also by such signs as "jumping at the
least thing", stammering, or restless sleep. These
two aspects could be considered separately, and they
are sometimes classified as "personality deviations"
to express the state of mind and "habit disorders"
to express the outward signs. But in dealing with
the subject as we are here, from the lay point of view,
it seems best to take these cases as they are brought
to the doctor or the psychiatrist : as the genus
"nervous child".

The word nervous may be an unscientific mis-
nomer, but it is widely used by the lay public, and
used moreover to signify a fairly definite entity, so
that we must perforce regard it, or its latinate and
equally unscientific equivalent "neurosis", as a

necessary portmanteau word, at least until the public and the medical profession are better educated in the subject of mental hygiene, or until another term creeps into common use.

The interest and importance of this type of childhood neurosis for the teacher, the school doctor, or the Child Guidance Clinic lies in certain characteristics of the condition, which renders it to a large extent understandable and treatable without very elaborate or deep investigation.

It is in the first place closely related to the *physical* sphere : to the inherited type or constitution of the child, and to various peculiarities in his physiology. It is often associated with physical conditions such as debility following infectious fevers, or toxic conditions from tonsils or disordered digestive function ; to bio-chemical states such as lack of calcium, or lack of sugar ; or again with a disfunction or inbalance of the endocrine system.

This no man's land between the psychic and the physical is still in process of exploration, and there is much to be learnt as to the more subtle modes of interaction between them. The physical aspect of neurosis in its more obvious features is the province of the physician, and is dealt with fully in text-books of pediatrics, but it needs to be considered here in general lines as affecting treatment, and is always to be kept in mind.

The work of Child Guidance has brought into relief the psychological factors of neurosis in childhood, and there may be a tendency at times to look for such factors at the expense of the physical.

The only correction to any one-sided point of

view is to adopt a psycho-biological approach, which considers the child as a complete whole, without any artificial distinction between the mental and the physical. From this standpoint the organism is considered in its functions at different levels, ranging from the purely physical to the emotional and the intellectual levels. Moreover, the child is considered, not as a separate creature isolated from his environment, but as forming an entity inseparable from the family and the social nucleus, in which he moves and has his being.

By means of this approach too, much useless controversy is avoided as to cause and effect. For example it might be said that the neurotic attitude of an enuretic child is an effect of the enuresis rather than a cause, and vice versa, but it would be more practical to regard the attitude, and the symptoms, as coincident parts of the situation. Again some forms of constipation may be said to be caused by anxiety, but a pediatrician trained in a more mechanistic school might say that the constipation causes the feeling of anxiety, or may be depression, through auto-intoxication. It is surely a waste of time to argue in this manner : the only sensible attitude is to discover all possible factors which have, or may have, a bearing on the conditions, and try to correct them. Most often a state of disorder of mixed physical and psychic factors constitutes a vicious circle, and what is required is to reverse the process—trying the simplest methods first and then the more elaborate.

One more point remains to be cleared up before I pass on to a more practical survey of the problem.

This is the question of inherited constitution. The case of two sisters treated at a Child Guidance Clinic may be taken to illustrate this point. One was a girl aged eleven who had been absent from school for some months complaining of choking feelings, and kept continually asking for water to drink. The other was two years younger and was consistently negative in her attitude—to the point of violent refusal of food and of other normal functions of life. Both were of the extreme asthenic type. The mother was largely to blame for the attitude of the first because she was inordinately preoccupied with disease, which formed the favourite topic of conversation at home, and was always taking her family round the various hospitals; yet she was the opposite to her daughters in physical type : plump and of placid appearance, though foolish in her attitude. When the father was seen it was evident that the two girls were his physical counterpart and that the second child derived her attitude from him, as well as her physique. Both children were considerably improved by treatment, but their physical type remains, although their posture improved. It seems that here the condition has been modified within the limits of their inherited type. They are still under observation three years later; the elder one is working at present satisfactorily, but only the future will show how they will react to other stresses.

It may be said, however, that such cases of clearly defined neurotic constitution are rather the exception. The great majority of cases of nervous children are less clearly defined in the physical sense, and are susceptible of change even in this respect.

It seems indeed as though in some cases the physical aspect and posture follows, rather than conditions, the emotional attitude. One knows the fragile, large-eyed, anxious looking, " delicate " child of doting and fussing parents, who is literally prevented from becoming healthy by the attention paid to his health. Such children, if removed to the ideal surroundings of a residential open-air school, may change very considerably in type.

The physical appearance of the " nervous child " has received a classic description in the work of Dr. H. Cameron, who pictures him as follows :

> His posture and his bearing are in keeping with his want of courage. All the strut and confidence which ought to be there have gone out of it. The muscles are toneless, the back is not held upright. . . . The whole body sags and droops, with rounded shoulders, receding chest and prominent abdomen. The posture of the body, lax and toneless, is an index of the mind.

This, however, is the type of the asthenic at the extreme physical end of the scale, and many children showing symptoms of neurosis do not fit the picture.

Some tend to be rather of the lithe, over-active and tense variety of physique, others are plump and lethargic.

There are, however, certain children who are obviously of a special sensitive constitution which is inborn, and they are characterized by certain physiological features. They react easily to fatigue or excitement, they are well one day and not the next, they get easily pale or flushed, they feel any little pain and make much of it. It is just these children who are helped or hindered by the attitude of parents and teachers, and can be greatly improved, in spite of their handicaps, by a wise regime of mental and physical hygiene. They are generally intelligent children, and mental activity will not harm them; moreover, they improve with age.

The effect of the parents', more often the mother's, attitude upon the health or ill-health of nervous children has been mentioned, and it is a point of such importance that it demands further elaboration. It is sufficient to have a slight substratum of illness plus an over-anxious mother to produce in the child a state of chronic invalidism and continued absence from school.

A few examples will suffice.

One little girl aged eight had a mild pyelitis (infection of a part of the kidney) which was apt to recur but yielded to simple medical treatment. The child was so preoccupied by her illness that she was constantly asking about the state of her urine—whether it contained blood, whether mummy had tested it, and so on. If one doctor was inclined to make light of the condition she was taken on to another. A neurotic mother and an obstinate father cling to the child's " illness " as though to a precious possession, and the poor child becomes thinner and paler and more unhappy in spite of all one's efforts.

Another girl was described by the mother as having had " rheumatism, diabetes, pneumonia four times, and enuresis ". At a residential open-air school the child showed no symptoms and was perfectly well. Another was having "turns" which resembled minor epilepsy, but on removal from home these stopped completely. Many more examples could be given, but it is obvious that to assess the reality of an " illness "—where no serious physical cause is discovered—the parents' attitude must be taken into account, and the severity of this type of neurosis will be found to vary directly in proportion to the amount of parental fuss devoted to it.

This type of invalidism which has, or may have a physical substratum, may be unwittingly provoked by a doctor who takes the line of least resistance, and takes shelter behind such labels as " nervous debility " or " anæmia " (the latter is a rare condition in children, and the pallid child generally has a normal blood-count). Its importance is clearly seen in relation to the child's school life. Absence from school makes it all the harder for the child to resume lessons, timidity enhances his scholastic difficulties, and reproof makes matters worse. An initial and inevitable absence from school may end in continual periods of staying at home, when the child has come to use his symptoms as a neurotic escape from what he fears. It is for such children that open-air schools, where all meals are taken at school, and the work is adapted to the individual child, are such a means of mental salvation.

The invalidism of the nervous child is again very evident in the case of some adolescent girls. They are generally, but not necessarily, of asthenic physique, and their history is that of the child with

" nervous debility ". They complain of vague pains in the limbs or back, their menstruation is painful or irregular, and they are often " anæmic ". Unless properly treated they turn into pathetic young women whose life is a constant struggle for health.

One of the most frequent symptoms of the " nervously ill " child, as he might be termed, is of course pain ; and the distinction between the pain of rheumatism and neurotic pain is obviously of great importance in the life of the school child. Pains which come and go, which are felt vaguely in the muscles rather than the joints, and are not accompanied by other clinical signs of rheumatism, are more than likely to be due to the strains of growth, or other causes, which are felt more by those children who are hypersensitive to any slight disturbance in their bodily well-being. Rheumatism, it is true, may affect the central nervous system and produce chorea, and any child who becomes more or less rapidly nervous in the sense of being restless and inattentive, and whose muscular control deteriorates, as shown, for example, in writing, should be suspected of being in a prechoreic state and referred for medical attention. Nevertheless, rheumatic infection itself is not among the major factors in the neurosis of childhood. A consideration of a large number of nervous children will discover only a very small percentage with a history or symptoms of true rheumatism ; I have found it to be true of not more than about two per cent. of a large number of neurotic school-children. The physical aspect of neurosis has been stressed, although necessarily very briefly, because there is a tendency in these psychological days to treat the subject as though the child were nothing but a complexity of emotions, with the constitutional and other physical factors playing such a subsidiary rôle as to be practically overlooked.

I now pass on to consider some points connected with the intellectual life of the child in its relation to neurosis. It is not my object, however, to discuss intelligence and the learning process, but rather the imaginative and constructive side of the mind. There is still much to be learnt in this field. Susan Isaacs, for example, who has had considerable experience while in charge of the Malting House School in Cambridge, states in one of her books: " The actual relation between the phantasy life and active intellectual interest in the real world of things and events is itself a profound psychological problem." [1]

We readily admit the effect of emotional disturbance upon intellectual acts such as learning, but we know little as to the effects of disorder in the field of intelligence upon emotional adjustment. We know, largely through the observation of Dr. Montessori, the importance to the child of the right materials and suitable environment for the child to " work " with. In her recent book, *The Secret of Childhood*, she carries her deductions much further, and makes remarkable claims for the effect of a Montessori work-room in normalizing neurotic and difficult children. These observations should be

[1] *The Intellectual Growth of Young Children*, p. 19.

taken seriously, for it is difficult in the modern world, especially in big cities, to provide an environment which shall be attuned to the order and rhythm of a child's mind. The knowledge of these truths is spreading rapidly through the work of nursery schools and clinics, but there is perhaps a tendency to supply the toddler with his needs, and to forget them with the progress of the child through successive stages of education.

There is too abrupt a transition perhaps in the Infant school to deliberate teaching of formal knowledge, particularly as the child is about to enter the Junior School.

Less and less as the child grows, is the imaginative and instinctive side of life provided for, and the senses of touch, vision and hearing are insufficiently nourished. It may be supposed that the country child, living closer to the rhythm of nature's seasonal life, will suffer less dislocation of his sensibilities than the town child, who is in some aspects overstimulated and in others starved. Means must be found, therefore, to provide artificially what will satisfy the natural intelligence of the child, which needs to be fed through all his senses. Every child is in some degree an artist in the sense of someone who takes delight in handling and fashioning material, and shows a sense of form, colour and imaginative creation.

It is a point of common observation that much of this appears to atrophy about the age of eleven, and it has been suggested by Mr. Herbert Read [1] that what probably happens is that the child's instinctive

[1] *Art and Society*, 1937.

life is by now rapidly coming under the sway of his conscience (or in Freudian terms the super ego, dominated by the principle of reality as opposed to the pleasure principle), and his creative activity, which is also instinctive, is likewise inhibited. One way, therefore, he says, of preventing this too sudden a transition and loss, is to encourage art as much as possible. But everything depends on how this is done. Drawing and painting of the niggling careful variety may be merely cramping. Let the older child paint freely on a large surface with a large brush, and you will see the difference.

This digression may have seemed to have little bearing on the nervous child, but it is borne out by the experience of the playroom in Child Guidance Clinics how much release may be achieved by the inhibited, anxious child, as indeed by any type of child, through artistic means.

An interesting example of a somewhat unusual type of neurosis helped by this means is furnished by a boy of eleven, of normal physique and intelligence, who came to a clinic with obsessions about dying, dread of going to school alone, and various compulsive actions. He was very confused in his mind on the subject of arithmetic, and this seemed to fit in with the abnormal rhythm of his life, if it may be so expressed. The usual methods of tracking down and treating the neurosis appeared to fail, and he was then started on splashing paint on to paper and making vague patterns in colour. At first he washed them altogether into a grey mess, but gradually achieved brightness and a certain coherence. At the same time he was being coached in number and, whichever means was the more effectual, it remains that he improved rapidly at this stage and is now apparently quite free.

The whole subject of play in relation to the treatment of neurosis is dealt with in another chapter, but the artistic side of self-expression has been stressed here, because it is an activity which can be carried out in the schoolroom, and there tested by experience. But the concept behind it must be understood, and it must not be treated as a lesson to be taught, but as education—in the sense truly of drawing out a child's power of self-expression (which need not be made a fetish in other spheres of learning !).

Play and work are, for the very young child, one and the same thing ; all through childhood play is a preparation for life and not merely respite from work. The best environment for this is the country, but lacking this the town child must be provided with something better than the street and the shop-made toy. Play and work in the right environment, with sufficient spontaneity and freedom, are preventive of neurosis.

The importance of play has come to be recognized more fully through the study of its effect upon abnormal children ; as has been so often the case in modern pedagogic or therapeutic methods, the lessons learnt from abnormals can be applied not only to their cure or improvement, but to enhance and preserve the normality of the rest.

To pass from this somewhat theoretical discussion to more everyday details, it is obvious that the handling of the nervous child in the classroom is an important matter. It need hardly be said that there is nothing so unjust as punishment, especially corporal, for a child who is too nervous, too confused, or too uninterested to do his work properly ; yet unfortunately it is still too prevalent.

A child may be dubbed " lazy " without any attempt at considering what this label may imply. It generally means bad teaching, because the child is not interested, and we should blame ourselves rather than the child. On the other hand it may mean that the child is not well, that he is getting insufficient sleep or nourishment, or that he is suffering from some neurotic trait such as excessive day-dreaming, lack of confidence, or mental inhibition due to emotional causes. Lastly but not least, his intelligence should be assessed, because the work may be far beyond his capacity ; on the other hand it may be too easy and repetitive and therefore merely boring.

It is, moreover, not only what the child can do which is important but his *idea* of what he can or cannot do. One small child was playing truant from school, and it was only discovered after some time that he thought that he was a bad reader, having got the idea from some chance remark by a new teacher ; actually he was quite normal in his reading ability. The fear of sums in the nervous child is of course well known and may become a source of anxiety by day and by night. There is something very absolute about arithmetic—a sum can only be completely right or wrong—and if some of the steps have been missed it is rendered utterly incomprehensible and mysterious. (Moreover, there appears to be some deeper relationship between emotional disorder and the sense of quantity, time, and rhythm, which as yet is not understood.) " Coaching " in arithmetic needs to be directed first to getting rid of the fear surrounding the subject rather than to further teaching. The child must feel absolutely confident of the first steps before attempting anything more complicated which will be only half understood. This may seem obvious, but some teachers do tend to become impatient at what almost appears to them as wilful denseness.

The nervous child then is generally a backward child and it is obviously important to find out by means of individual intelligence tests, which should be applied by a psychologist, how far this is due to inferior intelligence, and how far to other factors such as missing school or emotional anxiety.

The typical constitutionally nervous child is more often than not above the average in intelligence and, given varied and interesting work and an atmosphere of encouragement, will soon pick up, if he has missed some of his schooling. In fact, with these bright, restless children, it is a mistake to curtail their mental activity with the idea that they are suffering from " brain fag ". It is rather physical fatigue that will affect them, from sitting too long on school seats and not getting sufficient movement and fresh air.

The child, on the other hand, who is dull in addition to being nervous is harder to tackle. He may have acquired a feeling of inferiority and discouragement from the home environment and early training, and will often, though not necessarily, transfer this attitude to his school life. He may come to feel that school is a burden and a source of fear and this will naturally increase the vicious circle of his neurosis. There are in fact a few children of this sort in whom the fear of school, for apparently inadequate reasons, becomes such an 'obsession that they will face anything rather than going to school. The Authority may naturally suppose that such behaviour is nothing but wilful rebellion, and some of these children end by being sent away to an approved school. I have known one such boy who endangered his life by jumping out of the train when he was being sent away. Such cases should be recognized, after investigation, as being truly neurotic and treated by methods other than force.

It is natural that all types of nervous children should respond markedly to the personality of the teacher. The child who has been spoilt and coddled at home will hope for a gentle teacher and will react badly to a stern one ; nevertheless he will respond well in the end to one who is quiet yet firm.

The child who has met with cuffing and scolding all his life will expect the same kind of treatment, and will be apt to despise the teacher who uses no force. Ideas of home discipline will be reflected therefore in the child's attitude to the school, but needless to say he will come in time to accept and appreciate a better kind of treatment. To continue to repress the bold child of the streets by corporal punishment is therefore to admit defeat ; he must be won over by more friendly means.

There is, however, a more subtle, subconscious relationship, when the teacher is seen in the light of that parental figure or image which exists in children's minds. To the child who suffers from anxiety, the parent is emotionally pictured in his mind as far more potent and vengeful than he is in reality; there is a fear of losing his mother's love and his father's support, a feeling of guilt for transgression real or imagined, and dread of the punishment which he thinks will follow. These feelings lurking in the background of the child's mind may explain the apparently irrational attitude of a nervous child towards a teacher, who becomes identified in his mind with the image from which he constructs the form of all adults. The reverse side of this relationship is of course the attitude of the teacher towards his or her class, for this will be affected by the childhood pattern in which the teacher's own personality was formed. Revengeful or even sadistic feelings may still unconsciously exert their influence; the love of exerting authority may be a compensation for repression suffered in childhood—such is the warp and woof of human relationships. So in many cases one would wish that teachers knew more of themselves, or at least knew of the possibilities which psychology may disclose, in respect of their character formation, and the possible unconscious influences at work. There is one form of moral cruelty, happily rare, which may betray an unconscious trait of this kind in the teacher, and that is showing up a child in front of the others by sarcasm or ridicule. One small girl whose neurosis took the form of compulsive repetition of a bad word (the fact that this was not deliberate being perfectly obvious to anyone who heard it issue from her mouth in repeated staccato fashion) was threatened by the teacher that she would be stood on a chair for the others to laugh at her. Probably in this case the teacher was consciously aware only of her good intentions, directed towards curing the trouble. The teacher, in fact, thought of this child as being perfectly normal except for this " bad habit "—because she was not aware that the child was well on the way to developing an obsessional neurosis. This was explained by the mother's own obsessions and compulsions, which were due to her own experience of an unhappy childhood.

Another case may illustrate the manner in which the investigation of school difficulties by Child Guidance methods will help the teacher to understand and handle the case. This was a girl aged ten who, although quite intelligent, was backward in school work, and also suffered from attacks of screaming at night and sleep-walking for the past two years. She was the youngest of four children, who were all clever. The child stated that she was caned in a previous school for not getting her sums right (this would be monstrous, if true), and that her elder sister was held up as an example for her to follow. There were also indications, such as her dreams, that she was troubled by questions of sex. She also seemed more afraid of her mother than her father, and probably for this reason did better with a man than with a woman teacher. At school she was especially good at dramatics and dancing. She seemed physically tired and her posture was poor. Treatment was directed to all these points, and the reasons for her lack of confidence and consequent ill-success being explained to the teacher, it was possible to aim at encouraging rather than forcing the girl with her work. Suitable instruction in the facts of sex was also given by the Social Worker with permission of the parents.

Rapid improvement thus resulted, and the girl did herself justice at school.

It has been stated that neurosis shows itself both in an attitude and in specific forms of behaviour, such as habit disorders. So far we have been dealing with the nervous child in a general way, and something may now be said as to these more isolated symptoms. These may be manifested either in the more internal, organic functions, or by external, muscular symptoms. As examples of the former may be mentioned, night terrors, enuresis and food disorders ; and of the latter, stammering, and " tics " (spasmodic movements of particular sets of muscles, e.g. twitching of the eyes or mouth, shrugging of the shoulders). The organic disorders are naturally of domestic rather than school incidence, and are of interest chiefly as an indication that the child is in some sense neurotic. It need not therefore be discussed how far these disorders are physical and not primarily psychological in nature, as is sometimes maintained. The truth of the matter being that as in most asthenic neuroses they are partly physiologically and partly psychically determined. The interest on the other hand of the muscular habit disorders lies not only in the attitude of which they are an outward sign, but also in the manner of their treatment at school.

This resolves itself into one or two simple precepts. Firstly the child should be protected from too much awareness of the habit, by not being exposed to any occasions when he would have to recite or perform in front of the class, feeling that the others were being amused by his grimaces or his stammering speech. Secondly he must be helped and encouraged along general lines. These children often appear self-assertive and in a hurry to surpass others and get things done; in other cases they appear timid and self-effacing; the first variety are compensating for their feeling of inadequacy, and the second are accepting it.

The treatment of stammering cannot be gone into here, but it is of course as important to understand the emotional attitude of the child, as to teach relaxation and breathing exercises in a special class. Where possible expert treatment should be obtained, for although many " grow out of it " or cure themselves, it can be one of the greatest handicaps and a source of much misery.

There is one other form of treatment for these and other conditions of neurosis which might be mentioned, this is the method of training habits of the mind through the body by means of exercises, dancing and mime, particularly of a rhythmic type, such as Dalcroze or Margaret Morris movements. Combined with other measures, these activities are of immense help to the maladjusted child, whose inner lack of harmony and co-ordination will be

expressed in some way outwardly, for as Plato says :
" Rhythm is the expression of order and symmetry,
penetrating by way of the body into the soul and
into the entire man, revealing to him the harmony
of his whole personality."

One of the most interesting, and at the same time
difficult questions in the psychiatry of childhood is
to establish the reason why children respond in such
varied ways to situations which are in the main
similar.

Why does one child shrink and fear, another rebel,
another stammer, yet another steal ?

The answer must lie in part in the physical sphere.
It has already been said that the " nervous " child
tends in the main to one type of physique, with
certain temperamental dispositions, while the sturdy,
stocky child may be expected to be rather the
" difficult " child. In the sense that biochemical,
endocrine and other physical factors influence the
type of neurosis it may be said that it is " in the
blood " of certain children to react in a certain way.

But of this interaction of the physical with the
psychic so little is known that in the practical sphere
of therapy one must largely leave it on one side—
except of course for the treatment on general lines
indicated previously—and concentrate on the
psychological sphere.

From the standpoint of the orthodox Child
Guidance Clinic—which is the one adopted in this
chapter—our concern is mainly with the here and
now, with the child as we now see him, with the
environment of family, school and society as it

exists at the moment. To understand the present, however, we must go back to the past and forward to the future : analysis and synthesis. In dealing with the past history and the early origin of neurosis the whole family situation has to be considered.

In the drama of each family, of father and mother, brothers and sisters, endless diversity of scene and of passional relationships is possible, and we can only indicate here a few of the more obvious aspects of these situations. We know, for example, the effect of too close a relationship between mother and child, with excess of anxious affection on the one hand and of infantile dependence on the other ; this situation has become a hackneyed one, it might be said, through the term " mother-fixation ". An ever-present fear of losing affection either through the insatiable need for it, through parental threats, or through early experiences in being fed and weaned, give rise to the anxiety and other traits of the nervous child.

Actual deprivation of normal family life, either from the beginning of life or through sudden events of death or separation later, are more likely to produce outwardly a rebellious attitude to life ; this is more specially seen apparently where some-one else has taken on the rôle of the mother with insufficient understanding of the needs of the child : the stepmother of the fairy tale is often founded on fact.

One of the commonest origins of this real or fancied loss of the affection demanded, is of course a situation causing jealousy. This all too human failing which plays so large a part in adult life, not only in the sphere of sex love, but of ambition and career as well, is almost the rule whether in open and obvious, or disguised form, among members of a family; it is too well known a fact that difficulties of behaviour often coincide with the arrival of a baby brother or sister.

It is also a common story that difficult behaviour has started at a time when early spoiling was followed by reprimand and physical punishment. Often the mother will say, "I can see now that I made a mistake"; they have realized what I often say to parents—that if you give battle to a child you will get beaten in the end: he will cry and soften your heart, or he will get ill, or more difficult, or abnormally repressed.

Nevertheless it is a mistake to suppose that neurosis does not arise in a family which is seemingly as normal as anything can be: the forces which make for neurosis are inherent in human beings and their effect can never be foretold. Parents cannot always be held responsible, and are certainly not to be blamed, but simply helped.

The value of knowing the main facts about the past lies in thus being able to understand the logic and purpose of the child's behaviour, and it is often useful to be able to formulate in words what the child might appear to be expressing in his moods and actions, according to his unconscious, or at least unrealized, set of motives. Thus a child who comes to feel that he is no longer loved or appreciated and begins to steal, is acting as if he were saying "you don't want me, and you think I am bad, so I will be bad, and I will do what will hurt you most ". There is the well-known type of child who is said to be always trying to seek the limelight, but the point is not that he seeks it, but why he does so. Such a child may have been overpraised and indulged at home, and finds himself one of a crowd at school, so he must shine in some way, and if he cannot do so in legitimate ways he will take the easier path of extravagant action or naughtiness. Punishment will only make him feel more heroic and be therefore useless. There are other children who are not seeking attention, but are driven by the inner logic of their life to behave in such a way as to have the limelight thrust upon them. Such was the case with a boy aged eleven who was sent to a clinic after some stealing episode. The boy was " nervous " in the sense that he suffered from enuresis, was afraid of the dark, and easily upset, yet at school he was daring, rebellious and always mixing with the worst boys. He was the eldest of two boys in the family, the second being the cleverer of the two. His mother was a foolish doting woman, and had wished for a girl, so this boy had been brought up in a girlish way and played with dolls. His father was weak and kindly but very deaf. The boy wanted to be manly. He was good at sports, but his resentment at the petty nagging ways of his mother, in conflict with his dependence upon her, and his own " masculine protest " made him demand greater compensation than the usual success of other boys, and this led to a gangster type of behaviour. He was unfortunately not understood at school and acquired a sense of injustice and of revenge, so that in spite of partial success under Child Guidance treatment, he was finally committed to an Approved School. The success of such a school with a boy whose delinquency is essentially of a neurotic type is doubtful, and there is a danger that he may continue to behave in an anti-social way after leaving it, but some schools are amazingly successful even with neurotic cases, and the boy may learn to grow up more easily away from his home.

The above is a case where it is possible that the inner conflict required a more thorough and deeper form of treatment—a formulation in Freudian terms, and a resolution of it through psychoanalysis.

In cases where the nervous conditions do not yield to simpler methods of treatment, the causes must be sought deeper. It may be in the childhood of the parents themselves that the child's neurosis has arisen, since it is their attitude and especially their unconscious difficulties which are promoting abnormal reactions in their children.

A child aged eight whose sole symptom of neurosis at school was a stammer, was reported as being terribly nervous at home, and given to temper tantrums. He had been spoilt by his father, but the mother favoured his sister, three years younger, and he was jealous both of his sister and of his father. The mother showed a marked anxiety neurosis, and her history was that she was the eldest girl in a family of boys and had been thrashed by her mother and despised by her father—so she said. She had therefore developed an antagonism to men, hence to her husband and son, although consciously she thought herself fond of them. Treatment of the mother was necessary in this case before the boy could improve.

In estimating the degree of neurosis in children certain points may be kept in mind. In the first place, the complexity and duration of the condition; in other words—are the symptoms both varied and sufficiently serious to interfere with the child's success and happiness? The longer the duration the more serious the neurosis. In the younger child there will be at first, generally speaking, a diffuse condition of " nervousness " and the older the child the more likely it is to become differentiated into more definite phobias, obsessions, and other definite varieties of neurosis. On the other hand, in some children there may be periods of comparative stability and normality, with the appearance or recrudescence of neurosis when some new situation is to be faced, e.g. a change of school, or with the approach of adolescence. What is to be estimated also is the degree to which such response or attitude as the child shows are engrained as it were in his make-up or personality, or whether they appear to be incidental or superimposed on an otherwise normal or stable child. In other words, as Dr. Moodie has pointed out, the behaviour problem, or neurosis, may be the reaction of a stable child to an abnormal environment or to the wrong kind of training; or that of an essentially unstable child of neurotic personality (in which case there will probably be other members of the family of a like disposition), even to an apparently normal environment.

There is one other point in the genesis of neurosis which may also be referred to here. It was pointed out at the beginning that it is generally idle to talk of a cause or causes for neurosis. It will also be generally noted that in any case studied there will be several factors that appear to have a bearing on the case, and it is generally a combination or co-incidence of various events that precipitates the onset of a neurosis.

This recognition of various grades of neurosis in school-children has an obvious bearing on treatment, for not all " nervous children " can be, or should be, treated at a psychological clinic.

The doctor has to discriminate between those children where the symptoms are of a passing nature, or mainly associated with physical conditions, or where they are of a more serious nature requiring more elaborate investigation. Many can be treated by common-sense adjustments of routine at home and at school, coupled with such remedial measures as •ultra-violet radiation, physical exercises, or temporary convalescent treatment, not to mention glucose.

The number of nervous children who merit more detailed and special treatment is probably about 2 per cent of the school population. Teacher and parents are more likely to refer cases where problems of behaviour are in question, and these in fact account for about 50 per cent of cases referred to Child Guidance Clinics, while children referred primarily for nervousness, in the sense of fears and neurotic attitudes generally, only amount to about 15 per cent. This does not mean that there are fewer of the latter requiring treatment; indeed as the subject of Child Guidance is better understood, more children will be referred for the less obtrusive but more serious disorders of personality— the seclusive, dreamy, asocial children, from which future neurotics or psychotics may be formed— and fewer of those who are troublesome in ways which should respond to a good school environment and wise handling.

The value of child psychology to the teacher will be evident, it is hoped, from what has already been said, but a knowledge of the subject should be slowly and patiently acquired, and not be obtrusive, or used in too enthusiastic a manner; it is well also to avoid psychological " labels ". The chief danger of a little knowledge of child psychology is that one is too apt to feel that one must immediately " do something about it ", but, paradoxical as it may sound, knowing much and doing little is far more likely to succeed than knowing a little and trying to do a lot.

Discussing problems with the child or probing his mind may do harm, whereas a child can be made to *feel* that he is understood, without being told so. An attitude of detached if friendly interest, rather than a show of zeal, is always best. In the same way it pays better merely to listen to parents and give the minimum of advice, and certainly never to scold them. In this way they will form a higher opinion of your wisdom, and come to seek advice later, instead of being antagonized from the first. Patience from first to last is the keynote of success in dealing with problem children in the school, but patience of this kind must be supported by knowledge and understanding of their problems.

Finally the question may be asked: how can the school help in the treatment of neurotic children, once these have been adequately dealt with on the medical side and, where necessary, sent for treatment to a Child Guidance Clinic?

The answer to this may be summed up in the word *encouragement*. This has a negative as well as a positive side. It means avoidance of strain first of all, whether in discipline or work. Punishment for a child who is backward and apt to be easily confused is obviously harmful. Secondly, any efforts to push such a child on must be very gradual, and directed rather to clearing up the difficulties, than attempts to bring the child up to the level of the class. On the positive side, praise where it is merited has a very salutary effect; such children are always eager for appreciation. It may be a picture, or a model, or composition, which, though not objectively of great interest or importance, may represent a great effort or achievement in the eyes of the child. It was stated by an Austrian schoolmaster that every child has a " grand passion " and the discovery of this focus of interest or of a potential capacity, often unsuspected, may prove a turning-point for development in a child who is discouraged, as these children so often are.

It is difficult, of course, in a large class to give

special attention to an individual child, but it can be done in small ways.

The whole educational environment, however, is the important thing : a happy atmosphere, work made interesting, positive encouragement rather than fault finding—these are the things which make the school a place fit for children to live in, where the nervous child is helped back to health.

VII. PROBLEMS OF THE GROWING CHILD

By EMANUEL MILLER, M.A.(CANTAB.), M.R.C.S.,
L.R.C.P., D.P.M.(CANTAB.)

VII. PROBLEMS OF THE GROWING CHILD

BY EMANUEL MILLER, M.A.(CANTAB.), M.R.C.S., L.R.C.P.,
D.P.M.(CANTAB.)

RESTLESSNESS IN BOYHOOD AND ADOLESCENCE

IT is generally held with much justification that it is particularly fortunate for children to be nurtured in reasonably large families. The coming together of boys and girls under one family roof is alleged to give early opportunity for the development of social understanding. They learn to appreciate the differences of reaction and acquire a capacity to give and take. In fact, the whole gamut of human emotions is played out and modified in the family circle. The varying manifestations of love and hostility find their first expression in family life. Jealousy plays no small part, but devoted handling by parents who understand the love that is due to each child helps to modify this the most unpleasant of human emotional attitudes.

The parents themselves can distribute their devotion and authority over a wider field and the dangers of favouritism on the one hand and of unconscious neglect on the other can be neutralized. The gap in age between an older brother or sister and the younger members leads to some extent to the delegation of parental care and authority; and inasmuch as the strong ties which bind the actual parents to the children are in this way relaxed, the emotional life of the children is in some measure also healthily modified in intensity.

Whereas in the Victorian family a patriarchal atmosphere was the rule, and families were compact, self-sufficient and restricted, in our own day the social changes have made it possible for reasonably large families to cultivate an attitude of freedom by the admission of friends to the family circle, and for members of such families to form easier, yet profitable ties with persons outside. Each set of conditions, however, presented or produced its particular set of problems. While the Victorian family tended to create strong internal bonds, it led to an undeniable strain in the maintaining of them. In fact, they were stretched to the breaking-point, producing a powerful internal feeling of repression which led to peculiarities of character by resignation or powerful self-discipline. Strong passions which draw parents and children together may lead to correspondingly strong urges to break away, to find novel satisfaction in wider fields and to fulfil the deeper instinctual urges which cannot be wholly satisfied within the family circle. Within the mind, however, where escape is impossible, compromises are inevitable, but such compromises are not always healthy, inasmuch as they may produce neurotic reactions.

Paternal authority and its frequent accompaniment, a tender and crushed mother figure, may provoke, in the children, divergent emotional attitudes towards each of the parents. Independence must be sought in rebellion or in adventurous separation from home, where parental over-emphasis in excessive devotion or in despotism makes self-realization in the home impossible.

While the Victorian over-emphasis of parental authority has largely been modified as a result of the diminution in the size of families and the changes in family and social conventions, no one would be so unwise as to suppose that the fundamental human problems of the family tie have passed away. Family self-sufficiency has diminished, but with it the desire for freedom and self-expression has increased through wider and more varied opportunity. But it is doubtful whether the parents themselves are sufficiently separated from *their* origins, from *their* early emotional ties to accept with equanimity the new situation in which their children find themselves. But however much recent convention allows of new adjustments the deep instinctual and emotional bonds between parents and children remain for all practical purposes the same. Environmental forces now have a different angle of impact, they send out a freer invitation to the younger generation, but the forces within the mental systems of the young people themselves bear the mark of our long human history, and because of their depth they remain as strong as ever. There is, in fact, no dearth of cases of individual maladjustment which prove to us that within the family circle to-day, the small and relatively free circle, there are still sources of unhappiness and refractory behaviour which have their deep roots. But the study of juvenile delinquency which, it is alleged, has increased of late, demonstrates some interesting facts as to the causes of maladjustment which end in anti-social behaviour. Many cases of juvenile instability are due to deep-seated psychological causes which only exploration of the unconscious mind will reveal, yet there are clear and manifest factors which explain some forms of anti-social behaviour. It has been found that running away from home on the part of boys takes place at periods when there has been radical changes in family relationships. Of a series of 500 cases of this kind, 55 per cent. of the boys had never experienced stable environments. Most of them had lost one or other parent, the rest had divorced parents or step-parents. Nearly all of them had run away alone and not in the company of others, although they may have joined others in the same plight or had fallen in with evil company. Trouble at school only claimed a comparatively small number of this group. Loveless homes or homes where cruelty or injustice reigned were obviously places to escape from. The basic incentives to self-preservation and self-respect were jeopardized because of this loveless state in which they had been living. Dependence upon parental love yields a feeling of security, and in the absence of this love the unsupported victim takes refuge in flight which is biologically a perfectly normal reaction to danger. It has been said with much truth that society tends to protect the parents rather than the child in such cases, since the first move of the law is to sympathize with the parents who have unmanageable children, although it requires but a slight inquiry to discover that in most cases the family atmosphere had become too vitiated for the child and adolescent to breathe freely. While most of these cases spring from the families of the poor, we must not deceive ourselves into thinking that the comfortable classes have not experienced problems of the same kind. The burden of these remarks is to prove that without stable home relationships there is in the majority of cases no promise of individual mental stability from which social sense can develop. Behind every picture of gross family disruption there lies the more sinister problem of the psychological maladjustment in the minds of the parents themselves. In the same way as it takes two to make a quarrel, so too it can be said that restless children develop from parents who are not adjusted to one another. The parents eat sour grapes and the children's teeth are set on edge.

Running away is merely one form of childhood restlessness. Pilfering and stealing are other forms, even more common. Such acts may be directed against the parents overtly as well as against society. Very young children, for example, will show their stealing propensities only by stealing from their parents; the older child and the adolescent has a wider field in which to operate and he or she steals from school, shops, slot-machines, etc. It is extraordinary how frequently children steal, not because they have not been trained to realize the difference between " mine " and " thine " but because the article taken or the money stolen is a substitute for love which the child has not received. Sometimes, however, there are still deeper causes for pilfering and such causes can only be discovered by exploring and discovering other forms of frustrations. For example, in one case a boy was under the impression that his father claimed too much of the mother's attention and this jealousy situation led to his stealing only from the pockets of his father's suits; from his mother he stole nothing and it was only something intimate to the father which was taken. By entering into the mind of the child, by bringing home to him his true motives, of which he was but dimly aware, when he realized that there was nothing in the parents' relationship to one another that kept him outside the loving circle of the family, he was cured of his stealing.

The particular type of restlessness which is associated with puberty and adolescence must be regarded as having physical as well as psychological causes. To be precise it is evident that with the important changes in growth which take place at puberty and which are largely concerned with the maturing of adult sexuality, there occur changes in the nervous system which produce important alterations in psychological adaptation. For example, it has been discovered that there are alterations in the acuteness of the senses. Appreciation of touch and discrimination lose some of their keenness which the child possessed earlier in life, and there is some loss of co-ordination or muscular balance which accounts for the clumsiness and apparent angularity of adolescence. It has also been noted that acuteness in hearing and vision diminishes, and sometimes an increasing short-sightedness takes place, but despite this lowering of sensitivity, the feeling tone, as it is called, which is associated with all sense experience, increases. In fact, any stimulation of the senses, while less acutely appreciated is paradoxically more intensely felt. Pain, for example, is not so easily suffered due to this overtoning. This change is really not difficult to understand, seeing that the increase in instinctual urges due to sexual maturing leads to a greater excitability of that part of the brain which is connected with the instinctual life on the one hand, and that part of the nervous system which connects up the glands of the body to this part of the brain. Physiologically, therefore, as well as psychologically the child tends to react at puberty on a more primitive level. The type of imagery, for example, at this period may become as vivid again as it was in early childhood. This will account on the physiological level, as it were, for the vague ruminations and romanticism of adolescence. And inasmuch as the child is now becoming a sexually sensitive person, feelings become diffused and ultimately become embodied in imaginations which far transcend the narrow sexual field. From the point of view of mental economy and also from the point of view of moral control it is a good thing that this is so because it allows for the development of sexuality over a wider field, making possible the development of sublimations and these largely of an æsthetic, moral and philosophical kind.

When we reach the period of adolescence, sexual restlessness begins to make its appearance. The boy does not understand the nature of the forces that are working within him. Old discontents, hostilities and unsatisfied love well up from the unconscious mind where the unsatisfied urges of childhood have been up till now quiescent. A vague longing for satisfactions begins to be felt, but as no clearly defined object can be grasped, the boy throws out blind feelers which may grasp on to anything apparently which will bring ready satisfaction. Sexual interest will naturally be furtive and the fear of the shamefulness of an open expression of it will lead to substitute gratifications which may completely disguise the original motive. Crude sexual feelings will be translated into engaging and sometimes pathetic acts of chivalry, but sometimes the boy will be too shy even for this and may become merely irritable and hostile to the object of his devotions. The mother, the original infantile object of devotion, becomes unapproachable and girls may be given a sly glance and auto-erotism will be indulged in in order that tension shall be overcome. In some cases where a tendency towards sexual inversion has been present due to early over-toned attachments to the mother or even to the father, this emotional zest may reappear because normal sexual interest is forbidden, and there are ample opportunities for friendships with one's own sex to overflow into actual sensual interest. It is important to deal with such problems in two ways. Firstly, to see that a matter-of-fact sexual enlightenment is given to boys before puberty comes on. It is equally clear in the light of our knowledge of early child psychology that the peculiarities of sex-development have their roots in perverted sensual interests in the first five years of life. Passionate parental attachments should be dealt with as early as possible, not by scotching all sensual feelings or by giving the child a loveless early life, but by a matter-of-fact naturalness with regard to bodily functions. By the time adolescence is reached, the tendency towards romanticism in the child is met by a romantic response on the part of the parents. Some such tendency is inevitable if the problems that have gone before have not been dealt with. A variety of healthy outlets, particularly through group activity, will help to diffuse much of the sensual interests which reassert themselves in adolescence. The romantic feelings can be dealt with by allowing for the sexes to get to know one another on a social level and the aggressive feelings and hostilities may be handled by group games in which rivalries and loyalties can be cultivated in a social setting. The political, social and æsthetic dreams of the adolescent should not be greeted with smiling condescension or with signs of irritation. The birth pangs of an adult need as skilful obstetric handling as child-bearing itself, and parents and teachers must realize that at this stage they are not dealing with children any longer but with young persons whose intelligence may be as good as that of any adult and more often than not brighter and keener. The adolescent can therefore be met with an adult vocabulary, and if any explanations are to be given they should be presented without subterfuges and deceptions. So-called calf love is often treated as a joke, but an adolescent with an unmanageable load of affection should not be pushed too near the brink by ridicule, as there are many disasters which overtake some of the brightest children at this age.

In boys between the ages of eight and twelve a gang spirit is frequently noticed. Boys develop during this period of comparative quiescence a comical contempt for persons of the opposite sex. They band themselves together into secret societies, have queer codes of behaviour and occult signs of loyalty between themselves. They can be singularly brutal to one another, but the brutality is not just unalloyed sadism but an expression of the juvenile sense of social cohesion which abominates any creature that does not conform to the herd. These boyish practices are, as it were, experiments in social behaviour, and sometimes when boys band together and indulge in delinquent acts the delinquencies must often be regarded as forms of adventure, a throw-back to the prowling band, the manifestation in some measure of the hunting instinct. These tendencies can with proper guidance be turned to a useful purpose and in the play group and in the after-school club an admired leader may give these group feelings a profitable bent and goal. In adolescence the group feeling within the mind of the individual boy relaxes its hold because private urges become strong and secret. They are difficult to share because they are difficult even for the adolescent himself to understand. A bent towards solitariness is therefore not unusual and in some cases it can become definitely pathological. The adolescent therefore should be encouraged to unburden a little with some trusted person, so that the natural sociability of the boy can be given an opportunity for expression. In this way inner rumination can be overcome and the energies which might otherwise be trapped can be free for the pursuit of some loyalty, whether it be social, religious or artistic.

A condition which is closely related to restlessness in adolescents and which has always been most disturbing to parents and teachers and for which doctors are frequently called in to advise is that of Masturbation. At one time this activity was regarded with both alarm and disgust by the majority of persons, and even to-day there is still uneasiness felt about the problem. At one time when conduct and religion were regarded as inseparable it was held that any disturbance in the sex life of young people was a sign of depravity which could only be remedied by increasing the sense of guilt and preventing, through a variety of restraints and sublimations, what was regarded as an altogether evil practice. We have all grown up in a tradition which imposes upon us the strict observance of sexual restraint, and that while overt sexual promiscuity was strongly deprecated, solitary sexual indulgence was an unpardonable sin which brought its own punishment in the form of physical deterioration and various forms of mental disturbance from imbecility to insanity. This terrifying view is no longer held, but, what is more, it is felt that such a view can be positively harmful and in fact does produce such a feeling of self-depreciation as would cause the development of melancholy and overwhelming feelings of guilt.

First as to the causes of Masturbation: most students of child psychology now realize that sensual and erotic indulgence in bodily feelings are experienced by very young children, even babies. While complete sexual satisfaction is not experienced by the very young, states of excitability can be brought about by the rubbing of the limbs together and by excessive embraces on the part of parents and nurses. Sensual disturbances can be encouraged by the child itself, but they are also cultivated by those who are responsible for the bodily care of children and to whom children become very deeply attached. Thus a mood and a disposition towards such gratification can be induced and to which the child will revert in times of isolation or when external interests are not forthcoming. Some children may therefore be predisposed to seek for this pleasure when more thorny paths towards satisfactions cannot be trod. Usually the habit lapses, but may take remote forms in the guise of fidgetiness at times when a difficulty has to be faced. Before puberty masturbation is incomplete and is certainly a component in thumb-sucking, nose-picking, nail-biting, the picking of clothes and other repetitive acts which have a painful element in them as well as a gratifying element. It is likely that the combination of pleasure and pain is due to the necessity to punish oneself at the same time as gratification is sought. In later boyhood the act becomes more genital in character through teaching by other boys. Sometimes it is thinly disguised in such strenuous but sensually gratifying occupations as tree-climbing and rope-climbing, but inasmuch as these are healthy exercises, which have a real goal, the sensual satisfaction accompanying them need on the whole be overlooked.

With the advent of puberty, when sexual development is maturing, the pressure of new sensations will inevitably cause a focusing of the mind on the sexual parts of the body, and where there has already been a foretaste from earlier experience or from early conflicts of sensual indulgence, there will arise mental images and thoughts which increase the tension to such a degree that relief will be sought. Such erotic thoughts as occur will be stimulated by books and pictures which render concrete these thoughts. It is interesting to note that observers have found that the further these erotic pictures and books are removed from reality, the more they are dressed in semi-romantic garb, the more stimulating they will be. Straightforward physiological expositions of sex and procreation are less likely to disturb than are the erotically draped subjects. Of course in some cases where the boy has already been predisposed to show a distorted interest in sex and birth, even an enlightened exposition on the subject will prove equally disturbing.

Coming to more specific and individual causes of the habit, it must be said that boys who have developed strong but prohibited attachments to their parents or to sisters are much more likely to fall victims to the habit than those who have long before puberty freed themselves from these types of attachment. There are, of course, certain constitutional types who are more prone than others. For example, the quiet, introspective youth with a strong imagination, self-absorbed, may seek inner satisfactions from his own mind and from his own body, whereas the boy who turns his mind outwards and enjoys the muscular life of romping and group games will have dissipated his energies and his feelings too over the whole of his body, and the interest in the sensual feelings will have passed over into some object or in the attainment of an external goal. But we must not allow ourselves to make too sharp a type distinction, for whereas the habit may take one form in the first group, it may assume a different shape in the latter. All will depend upon the previous history of the boy and upon the possibilities he finds for external satisfaction.

The general effects of masturbation seem to be more mental than physical. Its physical effects are not nearly as alarming as some imagine. In fact, in a boy enjoying good health the effects are negligible. The mental outcome, however, is admittedly not to be underestimated, but it should be definitely stated that masturbation is more often than not the result rather than the cause of some emotional peculiarity. These have already been dealt with and it would be only right to speak about the vicious circle that is set up. A boy who, through introspectiveness and isolation, runs to masturbation to reduce tension or to satisfy some deep but prohibited longing, is likely to increase his isolation and his loneliness. He is sometimes dimly aware, and sometimes clearly aware, that what he is doing to the sexual parts of his body is forbidden, or has been forbidden, and that he must not only satisfy himself in secret, but that the secret must be kept. He therefore becomes secretive, not only about this, but about other things too. He must cover up all traces of the act and must fortify himself against discovery. He therefore becomes self-sufficient, inasmuch as the act is self-sufficient, and he may become aloof, suspicious, critical and even irritable. And furthermore, his sense of guilt may render him gloomy, apathetic and uninterested. Periods of self-depreciation may make him pull himself together to avoid slipping down the path which he has heard may lead to such evil consequences. He therefore makes good resolutions, turns to pious books, fortifies himself with religion to such an extent that his aloofness encourages him to cultivate moral priggishness. But unfortunately the cycle is repeated and the habit reasserts itself. In some cases, however, the inner moral censorship may be so strong that the boy will do anything rather than repeat the act. In such cases indirect satisfaction will be obtained through the outbreak of some form of delinquency. One boy, for example, admitted that acts of stealing only took place when he denied himself the pleasure of masturbation. In this particular case setting fire to things or the desire so to do became a compulsion. Sometimes, where no indirect satisfaction is obtainable and the act is repeated, the boy feels that his moral stamina is weakening and he loses all self-respect and becomes unable to meet people and to carry on his work. This form of preoccupation may have a deleterious effect upon intellectual work. An appreciable number of boys, who have been hitherto bright, begin to fall off at school. They become dreamy and apathetic and the teachers wonder whether it is sheer laziness and carelessness that has occasioned such poor output.

It is obvious that treatment of the condition should be directed not towards the isolated symptom but towards the whole personality. Moral exhortation is only calculated to increase the sense of guilt and to dig in a sense of moral inferiority which has probably already taken root. If general measures alone can be adopted, they should be designed firstly to increase the boy's self-respect, not by the condemnation of the act, but by encouraging the boy to make the best of such qualities as he possesses, to make him feel that his teachers and parents are interested in him as a person and ready to listen to and to interpret his problems. Every effort should be made to obtain a clear history of the boy's mental development, particularly on the emotional side. All sense of guilt should be eliminated, and while he should be encouraged to enjoy the group life of his school, the history of his affections should be looked into in order to ascertain how they have been deflected from an objective path. It must be made clear to him through this history that his thwarted affections have made him turn to himself for satisfaction and that no happiness can be obtained unless feelings are thrown outwards and not inwards. Where the boy presents a wider neurotic problem, or where there are indications that his character is developing on peculiar lines—for example, along lines of excessive loneliness or delinquency—he should be treated by psychological means and the parents and teachers should be made to co-operate sympathetically in such treatment.

It would be interesting to quote two instructive examples of disorders in adolescence which show the effects of emotional upheaval upon both intellectual output and social adaptability. A boy aged sixteen had been developing feelings of acute hostility towards his parents accompanied by periods of restlessness and anxiety. He was an only son of middle-class parents who themselves showed no signs of lack of emotional balance, although they had on their own admission expended much love and devotion on their son. He was always a quiet lad, studious but without any outstanding mental qualities beyond a slow and relentless persistence in all tasks he undertook. In the course of treatment the deep hostility which he had for his parents was traced back to a number of fantasies, which he had developed in early childhood in connection with his parents ; and it was further disclosed that under his recent emotional storms a great deal of sexual misunderstandings and misinterpretations were active. His ability to speak freely of these misunderstandings and to ventilate early imaginary experiences with regard to his parents reduced his mental tension in a striking degree. From a reserved and bewildered adolescent, shy and anti-social, he has become a contented and happy youth. His anxieties with regard to his parents have largely disappeared. He has now become free to make social contacts, and where before his interest in the opposite sex was fearful and furtive, he has developed a common-sense and healthy interest in girls of his own age. And what has proved most valuable for his intellectual development has been his freedom to pursue his scholastic and university career with enthusiasm and with ease. In fact, his intellectual output has increased so much that he has been able to achieve a university scholarship, whereas two years ago he was not considered sufficiently stable to stand an intensive course of study.

The second example is that of a boy of the same age who called for treatment because he had become so bewildered that he felt that he had lost all contact with the world around him. A veil appeared to have descended between him and other people ; not only could he not understand them, but he felt sure that they could not understand him, that his actions were strange to them and had become the subject of cynical comment. In his retreat from the world he had begun to develop philosophic doubts which passed on to bizarre speculations as to the nature of the universe and the mysteries of human conduct. On each visit he would come with a notebook in which he had dotted down all the doubts he had experienced in the previous day or two. They were couched in turgid language, which he himself did not clearly understand, but he seemed to derive some fleeting comfort by crystallizing out his thoughts in words, however meaningless they appeared to be.

It was pretty clear that these speculations merely screened anxieties about himself which were much more concrete in nature than his philosophy would have led one to believe. Eventually, the pressure of the underlying anxiety became so acute that he became obliged to admit that he was perpetually harassed by sexual thoughts which he was quite unable to marshal into any sort of intelligible order. Giving him a sympathetic hearing, and freeing one's advice from any kind of censorship, enabled him to put order into his chaos and he became able to accept feelings which he thought were alien to him with calmness and good sense. He now feels that he can cope with his school work and that the veil which had separated him from his fellows has entirely lifted. In short, what he had been suffering from was an overwhelming sense of guilt which made him escape into isolation in order to fly from the possible criticism, not merely of his fellows, but from what he regarded as his better self. Here, too, we have an example of the effects of an emotional barrier in damming up intellectual output.

No study of later boyhood and adolescence can claim to be complete in the absence of consideration of the subject of sexual inversion or homosexuality. This problem has all too frequently been considered in the light of open physical relationships between boys or between boys and adults. This is far too narrow a view to take if we are to make clear the true nature and consequences of this type of mental development. Not only does sexual inversion assume a variety of forms, but it has more than one root.

No one is in a position to say what are the inborn or constitutional factors which may predispose boys to sexual inversion and to homosexuality, but medical psychology does permit us to say something about the emotional problems in childhood which cause abnormalities in subsequent sexual development. A detailed analysis of emotional unfolding would be necessary if we were to make clear all the hidden motives which produce abnormalities in the sexual life. This chapter cannot attempt to do this, but the outstanding points may be worth considering. Other writers in this book have attempted to show the way in which the child is influenced by the parents and how the child absorbs the parent figures into himself so that his ultimate personality is both enriched and hampered by this absorption. Experience grows by assimilation and the persons in the immediate life of the child are taken in no less than the food which it eats. A child deeply attached to the mother may assimilate so much of her character and behaviour that he may identify himself with her, so much so that all his values may become feminine in character and he may ultimately face the world not as a virile person, shaped in the image of his own sexual prototype, his father, but in the image of his mother. Sometimes, however, the boy's attachment to the father may be so strong that in order to win his father's love, he may identify himself with his mother and so win the father's love in the same way as the mother has won the love of her husband. In a somewhat more superficial way a male child, surrounded by a feminine environment, may express himself through the manners and habit of that environment and a wholly girlish attitude may be unconsciously adopted which may remove him from all male interests, with the result that when puberty is reached, sexual feelings are coloured by a feminine point of view. Gestures, habits of dress, interests may all be non-male in character, and the result may well be that when he meets young women, he shares their interests, enjoys their company and experiences emotions which are by no means masculine in character. The struggle at this period may take the form of an unconscious battle between acquired femininity and a natural maleness. In his relationship with other young men he may feel himself attracted to the virile prefect in his school, assuming an attitude of adoration and subservience and his mask of girlishness will be unconsciously put at the service of some other boy who may need a girl-like figure to satisfy the vague sexual awareness that this other boy is feeling. An interesting case comes to mind of a boy of unusual good looks but somewhat frail physique who was the youngest child and the darling of the family. Always sheltered and protected, he became most dependent upon his mother, but yet admired his father as a strong, distant person whose love he had always wished for but had never received. Since puberty he has drifted about, and without malice aforethought has found himself in the company of older men, who, to put it mildly, took a fancy to him. While there has never been any overt evidence of irregular sexual practices, he has been twice convicted in compromising situations. His tendency towards sexual inversion has become evident by the fact that he has been found buying cosmetics and bleaching his hair, and he has indulged in all sorts of falsehoods to cover up the inner turmoil in his mind. He has recently been deliberately seeking the company of girls, but they have always been girls older than himself and his attitude towards them has been one of self-effacement rather than of domination.

The active type of homosexuality, which is frequently a source of anxiety in schools, has another mechanism, but this mechanism also belongs to the early years of childhood. It is usually associated with a considerable degree of aggression, whereas the other type already described is more submissive in character. These more outstanding forms are not difficult to recognize and their manifestations soon cause trouble and are detected fairly early in their development, at least as far as puberty is concerned. But, if they are to be dealt with adequately, their first expression must be prevented in early childhood by eliminating undue sensuality on the part of parents and nurses. Common sense and frankness is essential in the parents' attitude towards the child's bodily functions and the little boy must in particular not be allowed to fear or to have any guilt about his sexual organ. Moreover, too strong an attachment of a male child towards the father may produce in a child a tendency to become lovingly subservient to the father, so much so that the boy in early childhood adopts a feminine rôle towards the male parent. On the other hand, strong identification with the father may in some cases produce such a disdain or contempt for the opposite sex that all love relationships are only established through the medium of male friendships. All boys have been said to pass through a period of homosexuality or veiled homosexuality during the latency period. Where the ground has been prepared by a strong father or brother fixation, the boy does not free himself from this passing phase and puberty may become a period of passionate friendships which may be an amalgam of good and evil as far as future sexual development is concerned. If the love tie to his own sex is sufficiently strong and satisfying at puberty, ultimate emancipation for the choice of a love object in the opposite sex may become difficult indeed. But inasmuch as friendships are desirable and become part of the boy's social equipment, they should not be frowned upon, but ample opportunity should be given for mingling with members of the opposite sex so that such natural interests in women as are present should be reasonably cultivated. Mothers in particular must play their part in this emancipation. Everyone knows that mothers are very loath to cut the spiritual umbilical cord which ties their sons to them and, though it may cause them pain to loosen this emotional bond, it is their duty as mothers to see that their sons are given early opportunity in childhood to turn their eyes outwards to more distant objects of affection.